Pumpkin Soup
and Cherry Bread

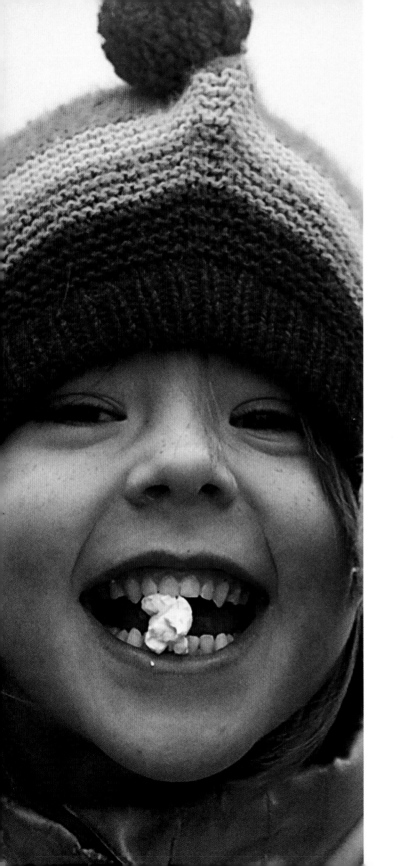

Translated by Agnes Broome

First published in Danish as *Mad og naervaer* by
Frydenlund in 2014
First published in English by Floris Books in 2015

British Library CIP data available
ISBN 978-178250-200-5
Printed in China through Asia Pacific Offset Ltd

Pumpkin Soup
and Cherry Bread
A Steiner-Waldorf Kindergarten Cookbook

Rikke Rosengren and Nana Lyzet

Photographs by Stine Heilmann

Floris Books

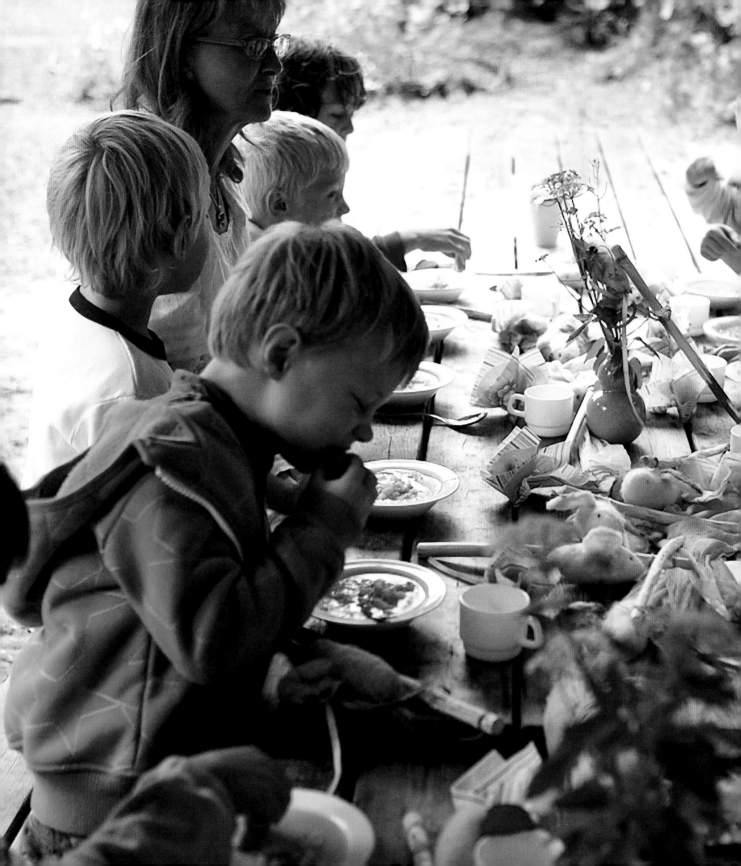

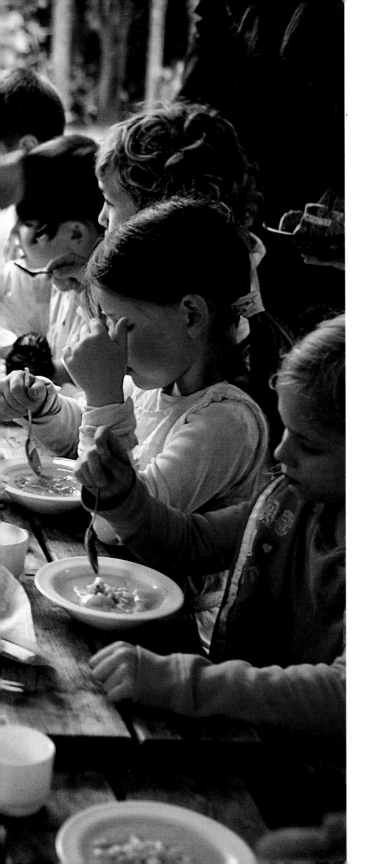

Contents

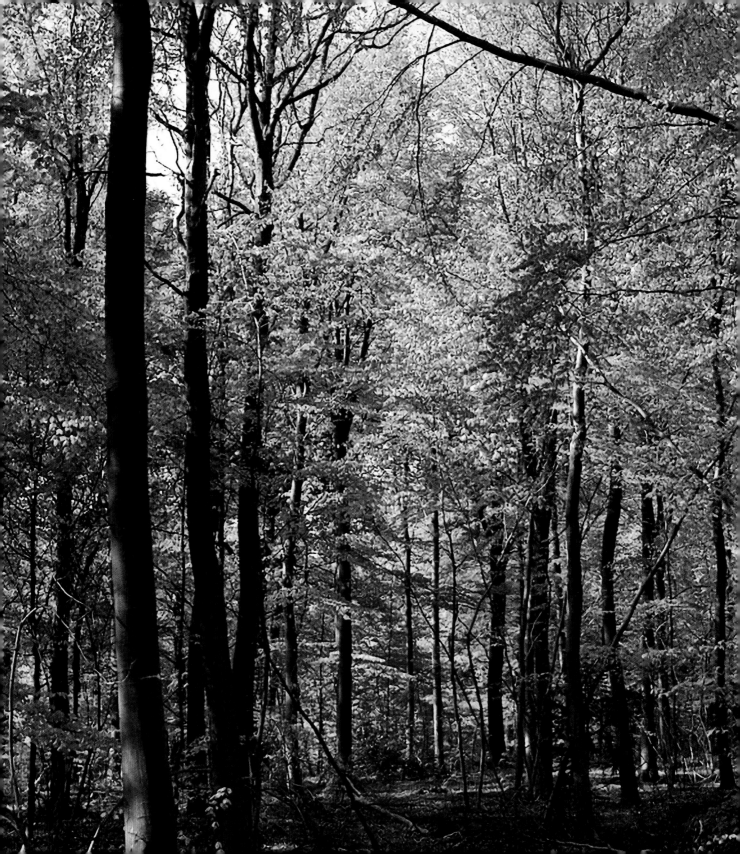

Foreword

Rasmus Kofoed

Rasmus Kofoed runs the gourmet restaurant Geranium in Copenhagen, which was awarded two Michelin stars in 2013. He won a gold medal at Bocuse d'Or, one of the world's most prestigious cooking competitions. He was one of the first chefs to put Nordic gastronomy on the map.

Shrovetide buns. It may sound prosaic, but Shrovetide buns (see *Fastelavn*, p. 134) were at the heart of my first experience of mindfulness and food. I was ten or twelve years old and I baked the buns all by myself. I can still clearly recall that I wanted the buns to be just perfect, baked the proper way. That required me to immerse myself in the process completely, to focus and be in the moment, to focus on each and every Shrovetide bun in turn.

On the whole, I spent a lot of time in the kitchen as a child. I was eager to explore the kitchen and my mother let me, for which I am, of course, very grateful to her today. My mother is and always has been vegetarian. That has shaped me, and even though I will eat fish and meat every once in a while nowadays, I always return to vegetables. There is so much to discover there, and the selection is never the same, changing ceaselessly with the seasons.

My mother also gave me the great gift of a love of nature. I had amazing experiences in nature as a child, which my parents' guidance made possible. Meditative experiences like fishing or picking mushrooms or herbs, experiences I've been able to draw on in my cooking. There is a unique serenity to be found in nature, a presence, which is a great gift, but which you have to practise opening up to. I can only advise parents to take their children with them to the woods as often as possible, as my parents did with me, when my mother would show me that I could, for example, gather rosehips or nettles to make tea with at home. Homemade tea is guaranteed to warm you more and taste better than herbal tea in a bag from the local shop.

My interest in nature also stems from a fundamental fact in my life: that I am a 'Steiner child'. I was raised with Rudolf Steiner's* pedagogy, attended a Steiner kindergarten and was educated in a Steiner school. Waldorf pedagogy has ingrained in me the significance

---

* Rudolf Steiner (1861–1925) was an Austrian philosopher who inspired developments in medicine, agriculture and education.

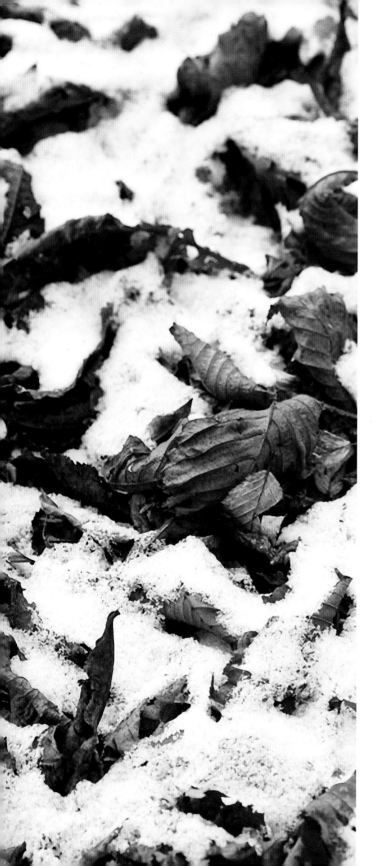

of nature – and of mindfulness, a dimension I am very grateful to have with me.

It goes without saying that the produce we work with at the restaurant comes from good farmers. I particularly value and trust biodynamic produce with a Demeter seal, which has been grown in accordance with Rudolf Steiner's agricultural principles. Organic food has, in my opinion, become too commercialised; too few of the producers put their hearts into their farming. The quality of the ingredients is paramount. It's what inspires me to explore the ingredients and create something extraordinary.

My favourite ingredients, however, are, of course, all the things I can find for myself in nature, such as herbs and mushrooms, berries and flowers. Nature may be my most important source of inspiration, and it's where I go when I need peace. I love foraging for wild ingredients and, luckily, I have a lot of people to help me find enough to run a whole restaurant. I incorporate nature into my restaurant as much as I can. It reminds me of the season I'm in, and seasons are important. There is a special kind of mindfulness to be found in working to nature's rhythm and using seasonal ingredients. Even when I garnish plates, I like to use something from nature, as a signpost, so to speak, but also because it's important to me to stimulate the senses and add more depth to the experience. It could be a smell that tickles the nose, or something to eat with your hands.

Without mindfulness something will always be missing, and this is true for the diner as well. It's in unity that harmony is created, and a dish is never much on its own. It takes two to tango, the chef and the diner. The chef must be present and giving, the diner open and receptive. When I create a dish, I try to create an atmosphere too. I'm not always successful, maybe because some people are more receptive than others. What for one person constitutes a whole story, with many layers, is to another nothing more than a meal. Presence requires openness, humility and receptiveness – and that goes both ways.

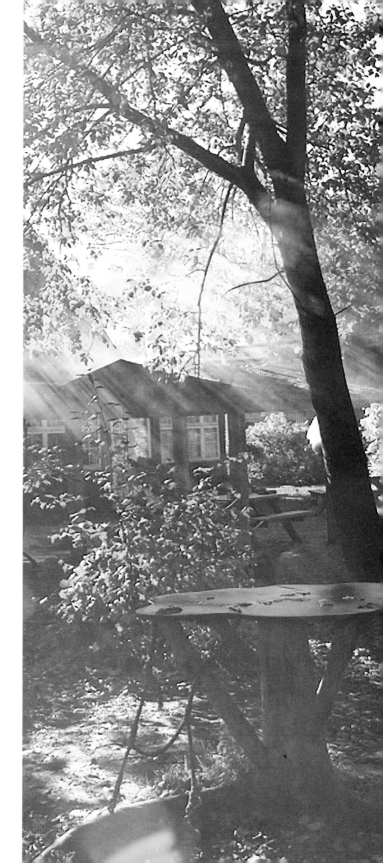

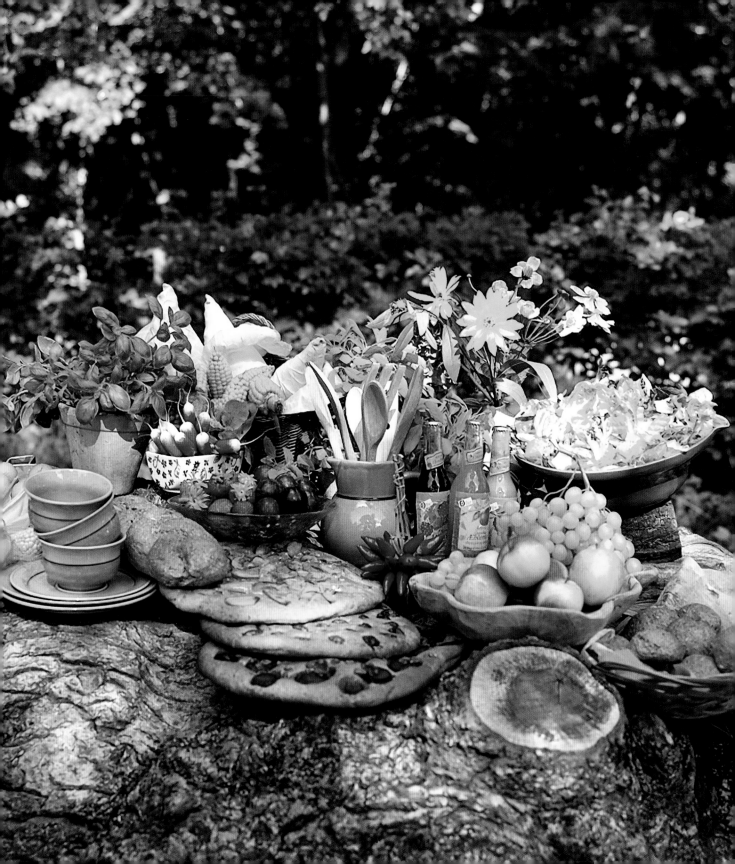

Introduction

The seasons have a rhythm of their own. The human soul can feel this life as it participates in it. Only when the soul allows itself to be influenced by the changing expressions of the year, week to week, can it truly find itself. Through this communion it will then feel strengthened from within.

Rudolf Steiner, 1918

How can I get my child to eat beetroot soup? Why will she eat it here but not at home? And can we have your recipe?

It was these kinds of questions from parents that inspired us to write this book. The Bonsai Steiner-Waldorf kindergarten is housed in a beautiful thatched cottage that used to be a restaurant – close to forests, beaches and parklands in Charlottenlund, north of Copenhagen. All year round we head out into nature and experience it with our senses. We cook over campfires, climb trees and forage for herbs.

We value diversity. Our children come from both central Copenhagen and the local leafy suburbs. Our staff is a mixture of young and old, men and women, drawn from every corner of the world: Denmark, Chile, Tibet and Ukraine.

At our kindergarten we have made the unusual choice of going vegetarian – and so our cookbook is vegetarian too. Milk has also been taken off the menu, as has, more recently, sugar. But, of course, children don't have to be vegetarian to come here; parents may choose to complement their children's diet with meat and milk if they wish. Our guiding principle is that we serve children healthy, varied food made from seasonal, biodynamic produce. This helps reassure parents that the food their children eat during the day is healthy and nutritious.

Choosing a vegetarian diet has several benefits. Firstly, everyone eats the same food. Secondly, by foregoing meat we save money, so we can afford the best produce and ingredients – and we can allow children several helpings if they're hungry. In terms of protein intake, children's daily needs are more than met by the protein in quinoa and beans, for example. We have invested in computer software to help us keep a running count of the nutritional content of the food we serve, to ensure that it contains enough protein and polyunsaturated fat.

The purpose of this book isn't necessarily to have others copy exactly what we do. Rather, we hope other nurseries and parents will make use

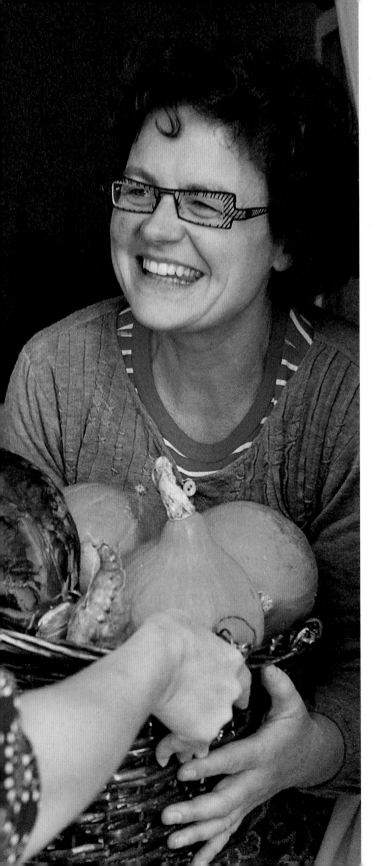

of our recipes and tips, as far as they find them helpful. First and foremost, we hope to inspire people to eat seasonally. But also to develop their food culture by planting a herb garden, getting the children involved, setting one day a week when the kids help to peel vegetables, and so on.

Food collaborators

Food has always played a central role at our kindergarten because nature, its rhythms and the importance of using our senses are so integral to Steiner-Waldorf philosophy. We use beetroots and red kuri squash, for example, in our songs, games and stories. Mealtimes hold so many opportunities for learning and development. Because it's so fundamental, food becomes a natural meeting point. The kitchen is also, quite literally, at the heart of our big house.

When Nana came to Bonsai kindergarten, after 25 years spent working in the restaurant business, she fell head over heels in love with the biodynamic vegetables from grower Solhjulet, the products sold by Swedish Goodtrade and the unusual and exciting flour range offered by Aurion. She immediately noticed the superior quality of our ingredients, as well as an openness from colleagues to further develop the eating experience. She sensed the possibility of an exciting collaboration with the staff, through which food could be given an even more prominent and considered pedagogical role. This collaboration resulted in new ways of thinking about food and meals.

And the food got more exciting too. From having porridge twice a week and eating simple pasta dishes, we went to making pasta with homemade olive and nut pesto and cooking exotically spicy dishes and soups. The children love it and eat even more than before. We also make what we call vegetable merry-go-rounds: plates of four different kinds of vegetables, cooked in four different ways, which help stimulate the children's curiosity and senses.

Presenting food to the children is a joint effort by the kitchen staff and teachers. We work in unison, food collaborators. Nana can't serve great food if the teachers fail to introduce it well. For example, it is important to taste new things, and our teachers encourage children to do so.

Food culture and culinary creativity are not part of teacher training, so initially the gastronomic skills of our teachers varied considerably. We worked together to disseminate an understanding and awareness of the importance of food and flavours. As an introduction, Nana arranged a blind tasting of various foods for the staff. There was also a crash course in the five basic tastes – saltiness, sweetness, sourness, bitterness and umami (a deep, savoury flavour) – and how they work. We're also developing several new sensory games for children involving flavours and aromas.

Children move with the seasons

We pride ourselves on using seasonal produce. During the winter we use a lot of root vegetables. When summer comes we play outside and need something light and refreshing like salads and strawberries. Our dietary and nutritional needs correspond to the changes in nature. Our bodies naturally need what each season offers.

Children live in the present. Rather than complaining about the seasons, they follow

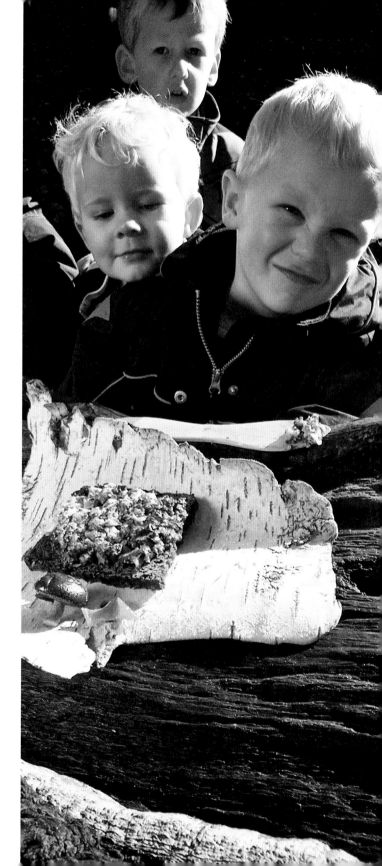

them naturally – so long as they are dressed appropriately. Adults often lack this connection with the season and just want the winter to end. But the message of this book is that life is fascinating and enjoyable all year round.

In writing this book, we immersed ourselves in each season, with the help of some of our parents. We have been out in nature, taking in each season and the unique energy and mood it brings. And we have talked about what each season offers in terms of natural bounty, sensory experiences and food.

At Bonsai we let the children experience the seasons through their senses. They peel the root vegetables. They taste seasonal produce. We arrange root vegetable displays so they can see the exciting and often beautiful vegetables that go in the hot, puréed soups they eat during the cold months.

Mealtimes are exciting

Our children all eat the same food, and they gain a strong sense of community from doing so. They talk about and share food instead of each sitting with their own lunchboxes. Mealtimes are incredibly exciting.

We want to show that mindfulness, food and the rhythm of the seasons can come together in a holistic unity that delights both children and adults – at home as well as at kindergarten. We want to convey the pleasure that comes from adjusting our lives and diets to nature's own rhythm. We want to show the benefits of making the children active participants. The journey from seed to plate offers countless opportunities for learning with your senses.

Seasonal celebrations are an important part of the rhythm of the year at a Steiner kindergarten. Each is associated with specific traditions – some food-related – such as the autumn festival, the lantern festival, Pentecost and the summer festival.

In August, children, parents and teachers take a trip to the biodynamic Kragebjerg farm, where farmer Henrik lets us say hello to the animals and help with harvesting. Many urban children think carrots come from the supermarket. We want to show them that there's more to it! After our trip to the farm we spend the rest of August threshing and grinding the grain we brought back, so that we can bake our autumn bread. We make half of the flour we use ourselves. We also churn butter and make autumn wreaths out of straw brought from Kragebjerg.

The autumn festival has its own lovely tradition. Each child brings a fruit or a vegetable from home. Then the teachers invent a story about them. It could be a story about King Carrot, Princess Courgette or the brave knight Sir Cauliflower. Children enjoy seeing the vegetables come to life and eagerly wait to find out which part their aubergine, cucumber or swede will play.

We encourage you to create your own seasonal traditions and festivals. In summer you might have a strawberry day, when you go strawberry picking, sing songs about strawberries and cook with strawberries. Autumn calls for an apple feast – for picking, chopping, gnawing, baking, boiling and telling stories about apples.

Routines make children feel safe

Rhythm is important to children because regular routines give them peace of mind and a sense of familiarity. Rhythms play an important part in

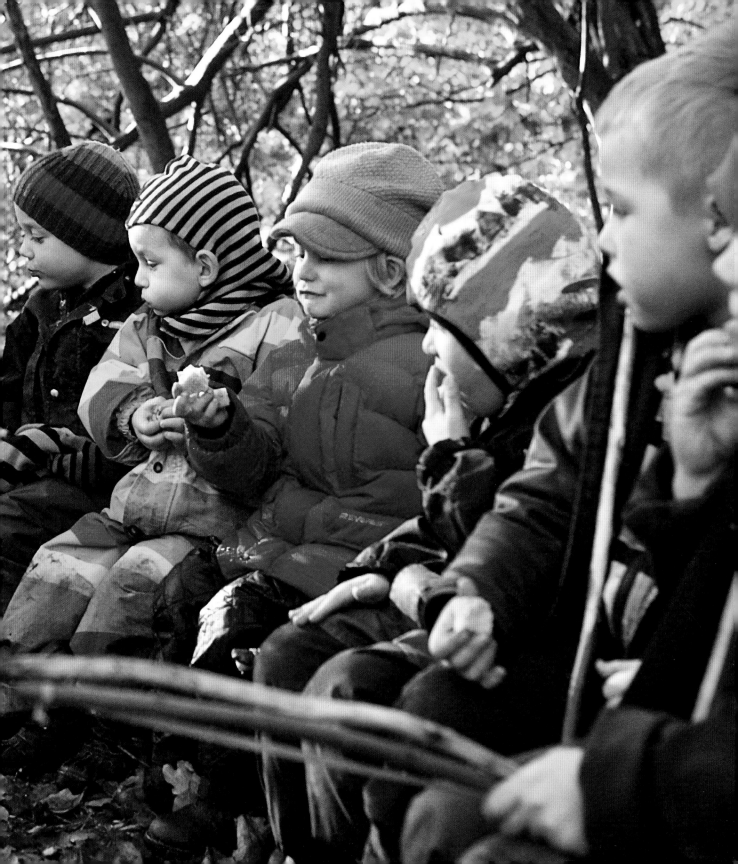

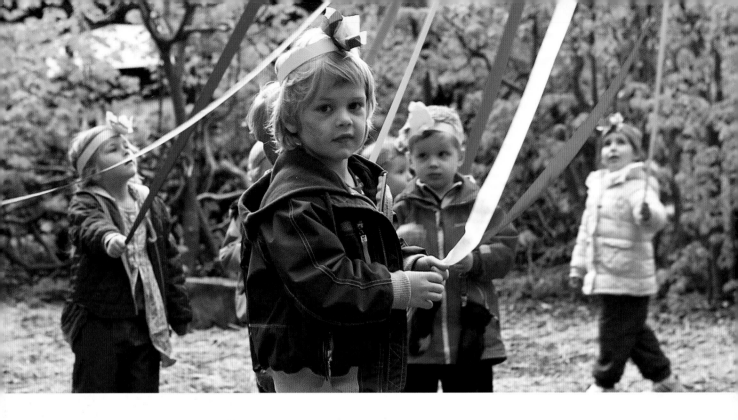

Rudolf Steiner's educational approach. He argued that children up to the age of seven thrive off a calm life guided by routine. They gain a sense of security from knowing that things will stay the same, which allows them the space and time needed to process sensory impressions. Many areas of children's development, for example, will power and imagination, are optimised when days are built around a familiar rhythm.

People are creatures of rhythm. We breathe in and out. We wake and we sleep. The seasons follow a rhythm that is reflected in us. We see this in our mood, energy levels and diet. When we eat seasonally we are strengthened physically and mentally and it's clear that our bodies are getting exactly what they need, just when they need it.

Rhythms at Bonsai

Years, weeks and days all have their own rhythm at Bonsai. During the winter we sing winter songs and tell winter stories. In the spring we might sing happy songs about light green, budding trees, flowers and birds. The whole day is unified by nature. It is holistic: they explore nature with their senses; they eat seasonal produce and they play seasonal games.

- *Monday* – we eat porridge with seasonal toppings, and the children bake.
- *Tuesday* – we eat sandwiches and go on an excursion.
- *Wednesday* – is casserole day. Vegetable ragout, daal (an Indian lentil dish) or vegetarian risotto will be on the menu.

- *Thursday* – is vegetable merry-go-round day. The children are served plates with four different flavours and colours. It is a classic and the children love it. And every once in a while there will be a new vegetable or a new cooking method, topping or dressing.
- *Friday* – we eat soup with croutons made from the week's leftover bread or some kind of marinated grain. The soups vary according to season.

At Bonsai one day a week is peeling day, which means the children work in shifts, peeling vegetables for the meal served that day. There is also a weekly baking day, and a sea day. During the cold months we light a fire in the garden and cook over it, and we do gardening in the summer.

On baking days the children are divided into groups. A few children and one teacher make the dough in the kitchen. They then bring the dough out so the rest of the children can help shape or cut it. We often bake over an open fire in the garden, then we eat the baked goods with fruit.

Fussiness is rare

When you take a closer look at the recipes in this book, you will notice that they contain ingredients and vegetables that are relatively unusual in most people's everyday cooking. Is it really realistic to expect modern children to eat *rygeost* – caviar made out of seaweed – or turnips and swedes?

We think it is. Our children do – happily – especially if they start encountering those foods early. Our youngest children gladly munch down broad beans and marinated chickpeas. Children who come to us from another kindergarten are often slightly more cautious. But as a rule it works

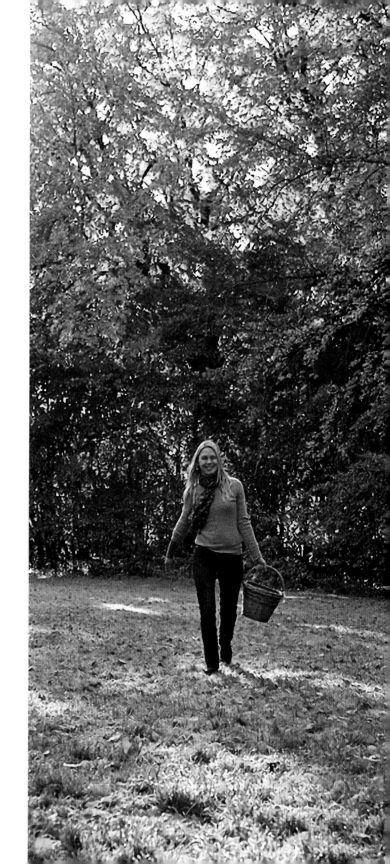

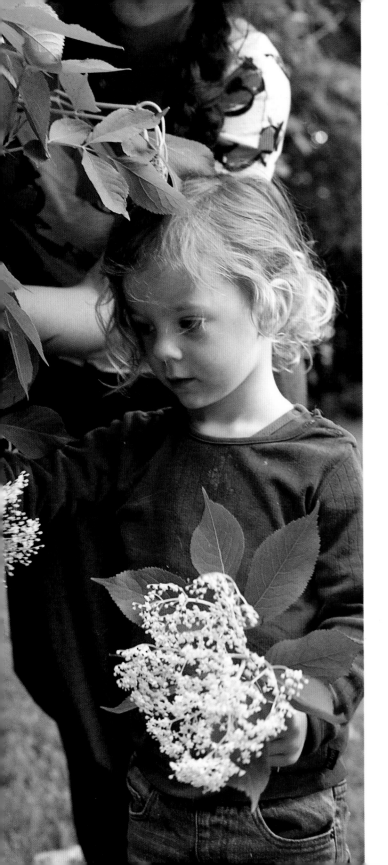

out fine in the end – because at our kindergarten food is part of a broader culture.

We believe that adults are role models. During their first seven years children mimic the people around them, so the behaviour of the adults in their lives is pivotal. If adults eat their food without fuss, the children will too. There is very little fussiness at Bonsai because everyone eats the same thing, and because the children have participated in the preparation by peeling the vegetables.

Mealtimes at kindergarten begin quietly without speaking, while the children try the food, then they can start talking to each other. There are a lot of munching sounds from the little ones, all round the room! They enjoy the food. Children are good at being in the moment – if you just let them.

We have some simple rules about eating: the children have to clear their plates. We are consistent about this. The youngest children often eat what's in their sandwich and then throw the bread on the floor. At our kindergarten they quickly discover that they can't throw food on the floor and expect to get something better instead. We also teach our children to finish what they already have before asking for more.

With our youngest children, afternoon meals used to take up a lot time. Now the staff have found a different way of going about it: while the children nap, they make little parcels, one for each child, filled with, for example, four pieces of food, some fruit/root vegetables and a napkin. The children get what's in them, no more, no less, and they love them.

Our biodynamic vegetables come from wholesalers, but we also grow our own in our kitchen and herb gardens. One of the reasons why our children happily eat vegetables, even the more unusual kinds, is because they are part of the

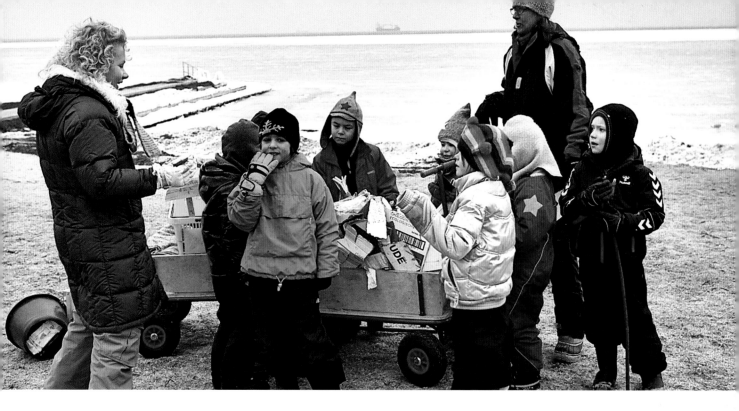

growing process; they can follow the vegetables from ground to table. They learn that vegetables can be part of stories, something to sing and act about. The children are properly involved with the food. One of their favourite things is chopping up a mountain of vegetables outdoors.

One hundred children can obviously not be in the kitchen all at once. But they can go visit Nana in smaller groups to look at her colourful vegetables, the exciting flour shelf, pots and pans and roaring gas burners.

Creating mealtime routines at home

"You've always been able to make my child eat beetroot soup. How do you do that? Even if I use the same recipe, she won't eat it!" We get this kind of thing from some of our parents. Part of the explanation is that we have a number of mealtime rituals that encourage mindfulness. We sing a song with the children before we eat, followed by a thanks-for-the-food song. It takes peace and quiet to enjoy beetroot soup, and children find familiar mealtime routines calming.

We would advise parents to introduce enjoyable mealtime routines. That might involve introducing a small ritual, such as lighting a candle, singing a song, or talking about the food before moving on to what everyone did that day. If there's commotion, if the TV is on, or if Mum and Dad talk endlessly about their work, children will want to leave the table and play. Children need calm and focus to eat well.

It's a good idea to have fixed mealtimes – early ones, if possible, before 6 pm, when children's digestion starts to slow down for the night. It's also important to make sure children don't snack too much during the afternoon, or they will have no appetite. If necessary, give them something healthy, like a carrot, to gnaw on.

Parents must also resist running back and forth to the kitchen to get things for the table. At Bonsai we make sure water, glasses and everything else is already on the table when we sit down to eat. That way, there is no need for adults to interrupt the flow of the meal; without interruptions the focus and attention remains firmly on the eating.

We are also passionate about…

Using leftovers in our cooking. Before lunch, we give the children a small taster bowl in their group rooms. If the food has been served, we are not allowed to reuse it, but it would be wasteful to throw away kitchen leftovers. Porridge can be used the following day to bake bread or make campfire pancakes – all year round. At a time when recession means tighter budgets, we are also looking at ways we can develop this thinking further. We make our own compost instead of buying it. We grow our own herbs instead of buying them from the shop. And in doing so we are creating learning opportunities that make environmental sense too.

The food we serve for lunch is always seasoned to contain salty, sour and sweet flavours. We try stronger flavours by using spices such as curry powder, masala and cayenne. The most important thing, however, is to add umami to the vegetarian fare, to really lift it. We do this by using mushrooms, seaweed, sundried tomatoes or olives. We can always tell how we're doing from the number of empty plates we get back! The aesthetic presentation of food on proper china or wooden plates is also essential to entice children.

At Bonsai we like to involve our parents. They have contributed to this book both practically and professionally – and we are very grateful to them for that. Parents often come to the kindergarten and take part in our work, and we cook together.

At Bonsai we like to forage for food. We take the children to pick elderflower, wild garlic, wood sorrel, stinging nettles and ground elder. We find food on our walks – rosehips, for example, grow down by the water, just over half a mile from the kindergarten. We put wild garlic in our soups and lentil patties. For our summer festival we make elderflower cordial to serve the parents and we pick elderberries to make warm elderberry soup in the autumn.

Parents can do all these things with children too. You might make a food trophy together out of seaweed, to encourage your children to try new foods. Head out to the beach and look for seaweed. Cook the seaweed and make a trophy from the leftovers to remind yourselves how brave you were to try it!

Our kindergarten has a magnificent setting with forests, sea and parklands all close by. So some might say that it's easy for us to live and work this way. But you can incorporate the rhythm of the seasons even if you live in a flat. In an urban kindergarten you can grow herbs in pots on the windowsill. You can take walks around town. There is nothing to stop you celebrating autumn in a flat by baking bread or making an autumn wreath or jam. Our satellite crèche on Amager, Denmark's most densely populated island, is in a flat. There,

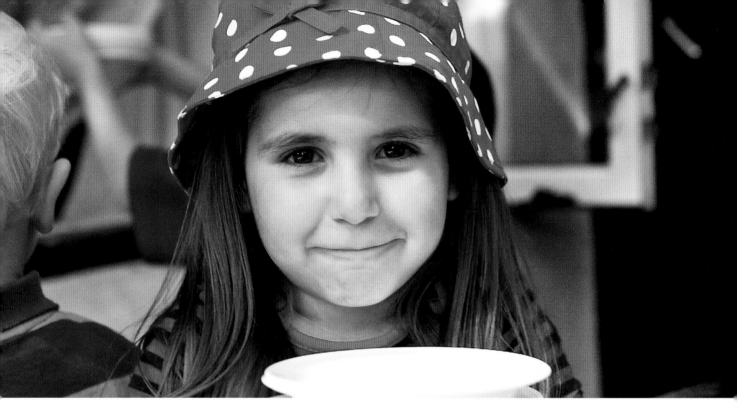

teachers and children immerse themselves in the seasons through excursions, sensory experiences, decorations, colours and flavours.

Some unfamiliar ingredients

You may be unfamiliar with some of the ingredients found in this book, but you should be able to find most of them in health food stores or online. Some of the flour types are unusual, but you can always choose more readily available varieties, such as rice flour, buckwheat flour or cornflour. If you are curious to bake with more unusual grains like *svedjerug*, Öland wheat or gluten-free amaranth seed flour, you should be able to find them online if not on the high street.

A note on seasonality

The recipes in this book reflect Danish seasonality, which will be similar across north-west Europe. If you are from another part of the world you will have to choose recipes to suit seasonality where you live.

We hope this book will inspire you to have fun with our recipes and ideas. Enjoy!

Spring

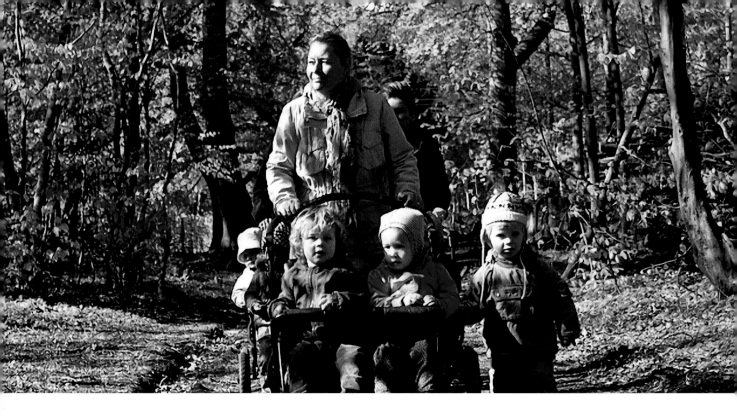

As we're on the verge of forgetting that anything can grow in nature, in the depths of darkest winter, the magic happens. Tiny yellow winter aconites appear, alongside snowdrops that grow in little tussocks with their white flowers drooping shyly towards the ground. And if you study the snowdrops closely, you'll find that there are tiny pale green stars on the white petals.

Spring brings a very special and much-needed energy after the long, cold winter. It's like setting off on an adventure; your senses are stimulated and it's almost impossible to feel gloomy when nature unfurls its splendour! What's more, children's experience with nature is influenced by our interest and curiosity; we should be open and trusting, so that our children want to learn more and feel safe making excursions.

In among the beech trees, the forest floor is slowly turning green, then the leaves on the lowest branches start to bud. Everything is ready, poised, and it seems as though nature has taken a big breath and is just waiting to really get going. The leaves unfold slowly and suddenly everything is green. Ready to eat! And beech leaves are actually edible and delicious in, for example, a salad, when they are newly sprung.

Our growing project

Children have an immediate connection with nature. Their lives are all about growing and maturing, just as the caterpillar becomes a butterfly, the seed grows into a tree and the tadpole into a frog. Every child possesses a fundamental, innate – and possibly even conscious – understanding of the concept of life; and adults can encourage and reinforce this through activities like our growing project!

At Bonsai we have built a propagator, where we can witness some of nature's processes alongside the children. The propagator demonstrates how light, heat and shelter support and aid living organisms. It helps children to learn about the sun's amazing warmth and the life-giving qualities of water. It is a simple expression of the value of protecting and caring for the fragile first stirrings of life. The plants are then gradually moved out into the garden, where they continue to be cared for.

The propagator allows us to grow kitchen herbs, vegetables and plants not normally found in our cold climate; the children can taste, smell and enjoy the rich diversity of the world.

The propagator is part of a larger project that includes the kitchen garden, cooking over an open fire and eating wild plants, all of which give children the tools to develop an understanding of life and an insight into the great cycle that surrounds us. An intricate and complex system can be made concrete, tangible, meaningful, simple and still truly magical for even the youngest children.

Growing tadpoles

Take a small glass and fill it up with water from a lake, catch tadpoles using a net, put them in the glass and cover. There are enough nutrients in the water for the tadpoles. When they've turned into frogs, release them back into the same lake. There is a lot to talk about when you're tracking the daily progress of tadpoles!

A few words about cultivation

Growing plants can be as simple as sowing some cress on cotton wool. Other grasses and cereal grains can be grown in compost in a bowl or a milk carton cut lengthwise. Edible sprouts are especially fun! You can, for example, grow mung beans or alfalfa. You can grow seeds on plates or dishes or you can buy special, three-layered germination boxes. A germination box lets you follow the germination of small plants. When germinating something destined for the herb garden, such as sunflowers and tomatoes, you can use old planters. Around Eastertime you can sow things like oats, einkorn wheat or spelt. Let children grow their own indoor Easter gardens; grains will sprout in early spring!

Playing outside

It's important to let children express themselves in nature and to explore, but all children are different: some are cautious while others swing from branch to branch in the tallest trees. Neither is better than the other and it's incredibly important to let children define their own limits. You must never under any circumstance help children climb trees that they can't ascend on their own. When their motor skills and muscles are ready, children will be able to climb up by themselves and stay balanced without assistance. The same is true at the playground with slides, swings and climbing frames. If you start getting involved,

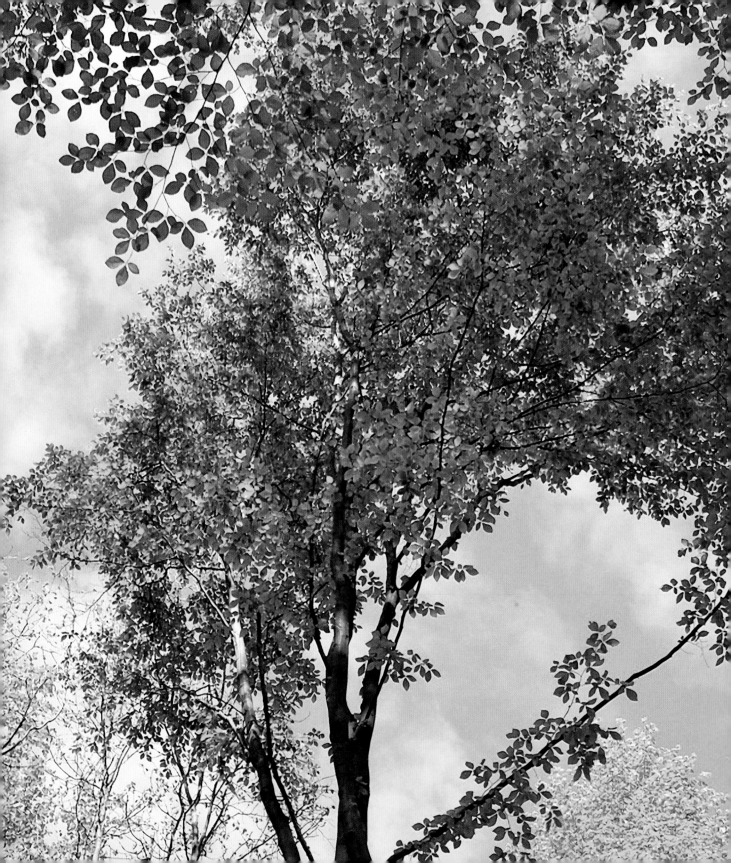

if only to help out, you risk children becoming dependent on constant adult presence.

Young children below the age of three should play on the ground. They will often play in a sandpit, and when they reach two or three they may begin to clamber onto the lowest branches. Three to six-year-olds test their own abilities and balance by climbing higher and higher. Some children may climb so high that adults need to keep cool heads and nerves of steel, but if they're able to climb, they should be allowed to. Unless of course it seems completely irresponsible! It's always, after all, the adult's responsibility to make sure there are no accidents.

Insects and insect bites

It is not possible to completely avoid insect bites. But if you stay calm, children will too, which reduces the risk of being stung.

If you do get stung, Weleda Combudoron gel helps. If you are prone to mosquito bites, onion juice can alleviate the itching. A sprinkling of sugar can soothe bee and wasp stings. And remember that yellow and other brightly coloured clothes, as well as sparkly jewellery and perfume, attract bugs.

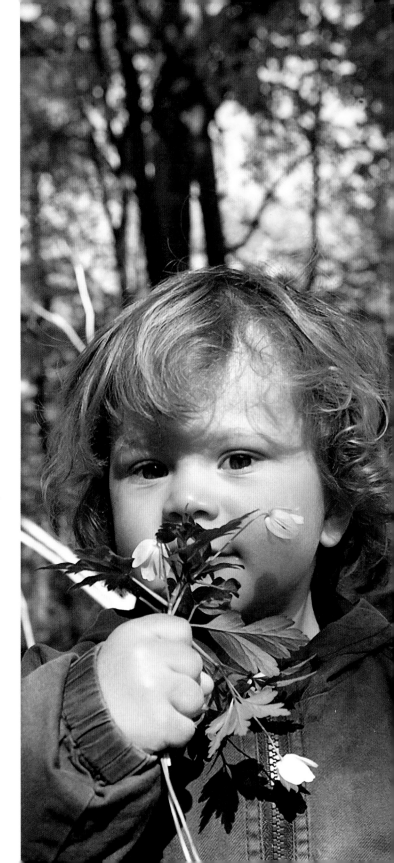

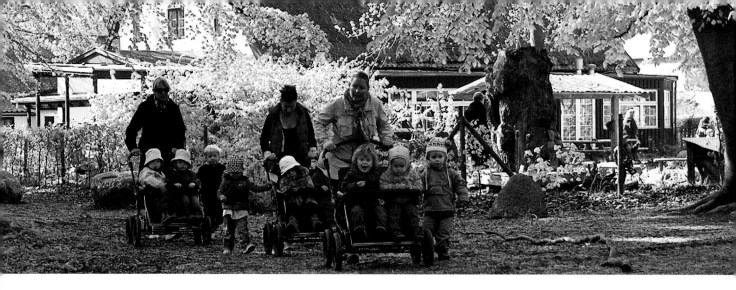

Rhubarb relish

It's wonderful to have a stock of homemade relishes and pickles in your fridge, and it's always lovely to receive them as a gift. There is something almost meditative about jam- and pickle-making, and it is an excellent group project.

Serves a family of 4
1 bunch of rhubarb
2 large red onions
4 tbsp quality oil
3 tbsp white balsamic vinegar
1 tsp herb salt
2 celery stalks
1 whole apple
1 tbsp finely chopped mint

Serves 40 children
6 bunches of rhubarb
5 large red onions
200 ml (⅞ cup) quality oil
100 ml (½ cup) white balsamic vinegar
3 tsp herb salt
20 celery stalks
5 whole apples
1 bunch of finely chopped mint

1. Dice the rhubarb and red onion and sauté in the oil.
2. Add the vinegar and herb salt.
3. Dice the celery and apple and add to the pan.
4. Season with mint, and serve on bread or as a condiment to main dishes.

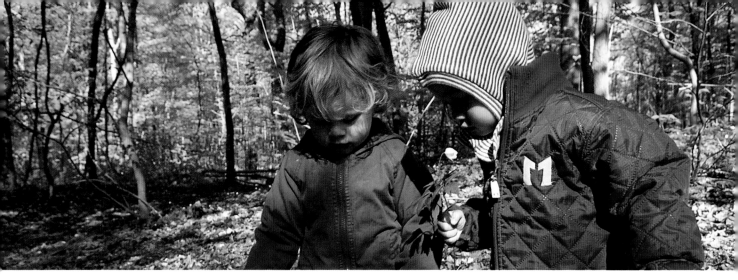

Rhubarb cordial

This is the ultimate spring cordial. You can substitute agave syrup for the sugar, if you prefer. If you do, use 35 g (1¼ oz) of syrup per 100 ml (½ cup) of cordial.

Makes approx. 2 l (4 US pints)
1 kg (2 lb 3 oz) rhubarb
500 ml (1 US pint) water
40 g (1 ½ oz) demerara sugar per 100 ml (½ cup) of
   strained cordial
25 whole cinnamon sticks

1. Cut the rhubarb stalks into 2.5 cm (1 in) pieces. Put them in a large pan with the water and bring to the boil.
2. Add the cinnamon sticks and leave to simmer for 20 minutes.
3. Pour the liquid through a sieve and allow to drain thoroughly. Then bring the strained cordial back to the boil and stir in an appropriate amount of sugar.
4. Pour the cordial into sterilised bottles, seal and store in the fridge. Bottles taken straight from the dishwasher will be sterile. Serve 1 part cordial to 3 parts water.

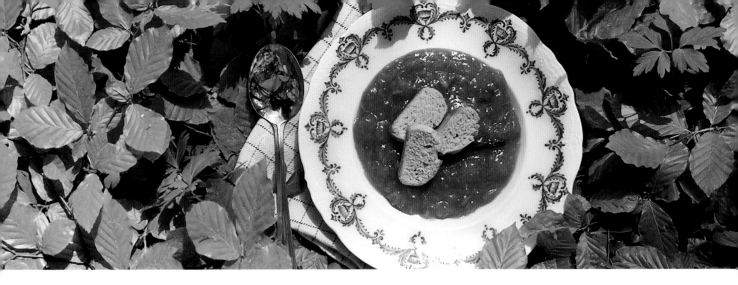

Rhubarb compote

This delicious dessert is lactose and gluten free, but you can add milk if you prefer.

Serves a family of 4
600 g (1 lb 5 oz) rhubarb
160 g (5 ½ oz) demerara sugar
½ cinnamon stick
½ vanilla pod
zest of ½ organic lemon
100 ml (½ cup) water or unsweetened fruit juice
2 tsp potato flour
100 ml (½ cup) water

Serves 40 children
4 kg (8 lb 13 oz) rhubarb
1.12 kg (2 lb 8 oz) demerara sugar
5 cinnamon sticks
4 vanilla pods
zest of 5 organic lemons
1.2 l (2 ½ US pints) water or unsweetened fruit juice
8–10 tbsp potato flour
1 l (2 US pints) water

1. Cut the washed rhubarb into 2.5 cm (1 in) wide slices and put them in a heavy pan. Add the sugar, cinnamon, vanilla and lemon zest. Pour in the water and let it simmer for 20 minutes.
2. Dissolve the potato flour in a little cold water and use to thicken the compote. Don't add too much as the thickening can be sudden!
3. Take the porridge off the heat and serve with amaranth biscuits (see below) and milk.

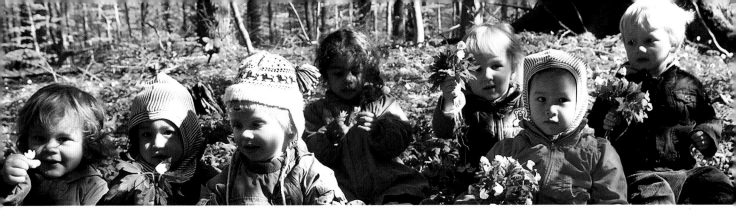

Amaranth biscuits

Amaranth seed flour is a new type of gluten-free flour from South America. It's quite different from traditional baking flours, but it's great to work with and it gives gluten-intolerant people more options.

Makes 60 biscuits
2 large organic eggs
150 g (5 ¼ oz) agave syrup
50 g (1 ¾ oz) coconut butter or melted butter
300 g (10 ½ oz) amaranth seed flour
300 g (10 ½ oz) rice flour or buckwheat flour
1 tsp baking powder
a pinch of salt
a pinch of ground cardamom

1. Melt the butter or coconut butter and leave to cool.
2. Beat together the eggs and syrup and add the fat.
3. Then work the flours, baking powder, salt and cardamom into the mixture and knead the dough lightly. Let the dough rest in a cold place for at least an hour.
4. Split the dough into 3 sections and roll each into a 30 cm (1 ft) sausage shape.
5. Prebake at 180°C (350°F) for around 25 minutes.
6. When the baked logs have cooled a little, cut them into roughly ½ cm (¼ in) thick biscuits.
7. Finish the biscuits by baking them for another 20 minutes at 150°C (300°F).

The biscuits are best stored in a biscuit tin lined with greaseproof paper.

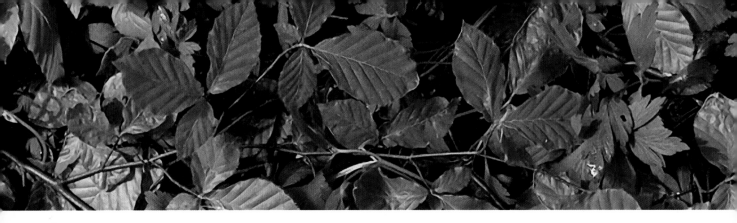

Turnip carpaccio

Turnips are beautiful white beets with pale pink skin. The taste is slightly sharp, similar to radishes. Some of the children were struggling to truly fall in love with the turnip, until this dish came along…

Serves a family of 4
approx. 250 g (9 oz) newly sprouted beech
  leaves, ground elder or other spring leaves
4 turnips
4 tbsp quality olive oil
2 tbsp white balsamic vinegar
1 tsp herb salt
freshly ground pepper
½ pomegranate
50 g (1 ¾ oz) pine nuts

Serves 40 children
approx. 2.5 kg (5 lb 8 oz) newly sprouted beech
  leaves, ground elder or other spring leaves
2 kg (4 lb 7 oz) turnips
300 ml (1 ¼ cups) quality olive oil
150 ml (⅔ cup) white balsamic vinegar
2 tsp herb salt
freshly ground pepper
3 pomegranates
150 g (5 ¼ oz) pine nuts

1. Toss the leaves with a few dashes each of oil and vinegar, and season.
2. Wash the turnips and slice them very finely, using a mandolin if you have one. Arrange the slices neatly in overlapping circles on a serving plate.
3. Make a dressing from the oil, white balsamic vinegar, salt, pepper and pomegranate seeds, and brush it onto the turnips.
4. Roast the pine nuts in a hot pan until golden in a hot pan and sprinkle them over the dish.
5. Arrange the salad in the middle of the carpaccio, and serve as a starter or light lunch with wholegrain bread or rye bread croutons.

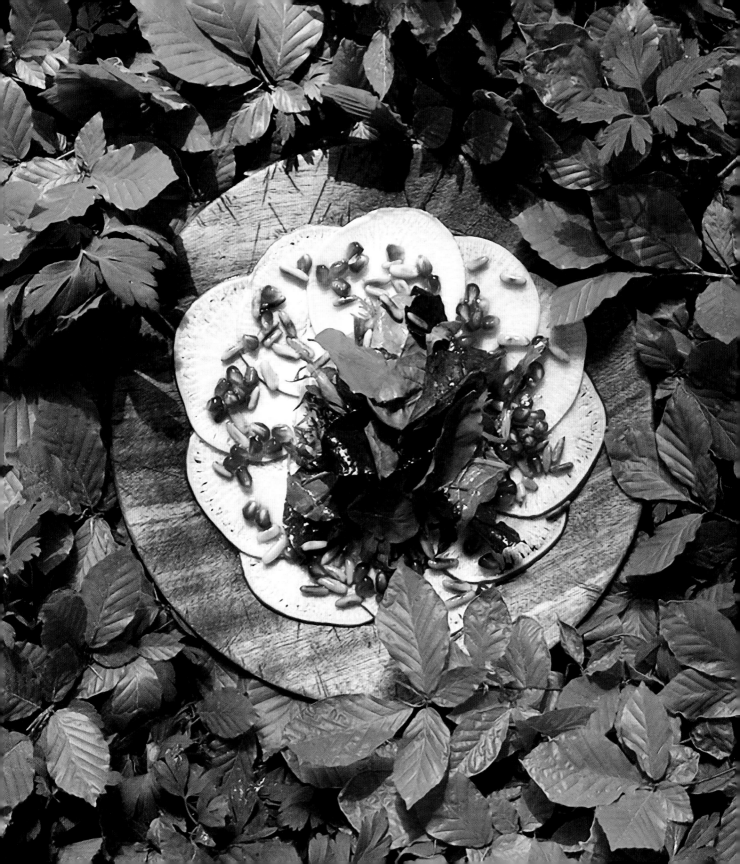

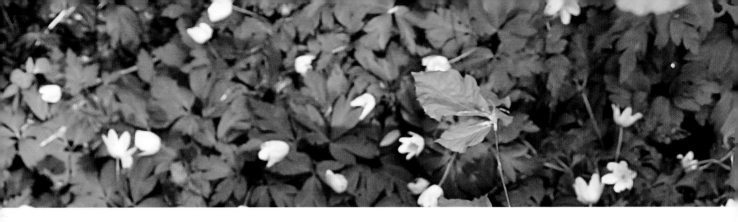

Crustless cabbage quiche with spring onions

This quiche is made with leftover daal. In a professional kitchen, for financial reasons, nothing goes to waste. The same should be true at home. Before buying expensive take-aways, have a think about what you could make from the leftovers in your fridge. Sometimes a half-empty fridge can be more inspiring than you might expect.

Serves 8–10

½ white cabbage
1 bunch of spring onions
5 large organic eggs
7 tbsp Öland wheat flour or amaranth seed flour (gluten free)
500 g (1 lb 2 oz) leftover rice, lentils or similar
1 tsp thyme
100 ml (½ cup) quality oil
2 tsp herb salt
freshly ground pepper

Serves 40 children

3 white cabbages
5 bunches of spring onions
15 large organic eggs
450 g (1 lb) Öland wheat flour or amaranth seed flour (gluten free)
2 kg (4 lb 7 oz) leftover rice, lentils or similar
2 tsp thyme
300 ml (1 ¼ cups) quality oil
7 tsp herb salt
freshly ground pepper

1. Chop the cabbage and spring onions.
2. Mix all the other ingredients in a bowl and add the vegetables. Season with salt and pepper to taste.
3. Pour the quiche mixture into a pie dish and bake at 200°C (400°F) for 30–40 minutes.
4. The quiche can be enjoyed as a main course or a sandwich filler.

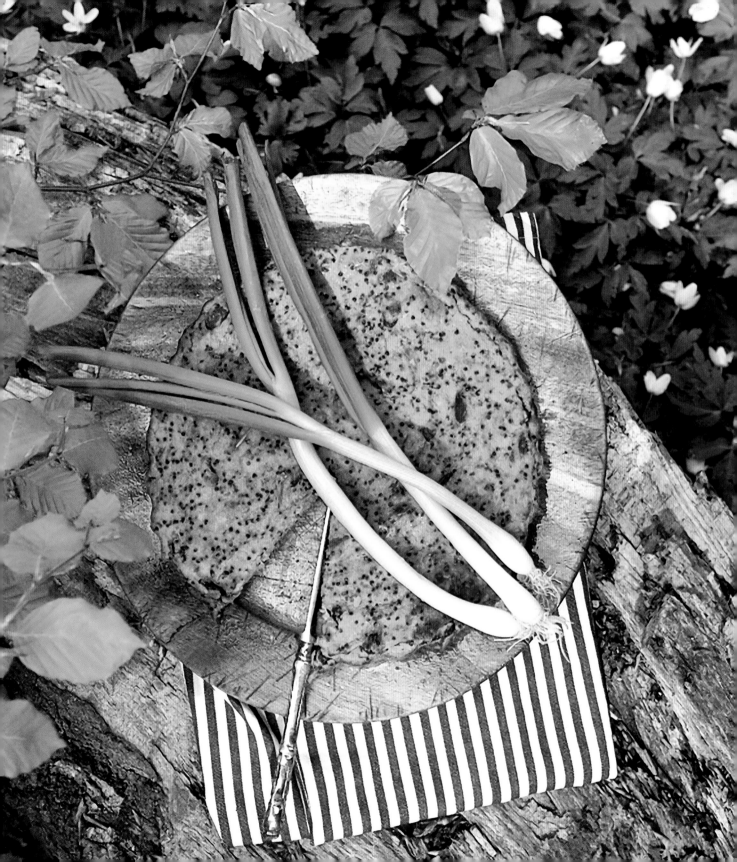

Asparagus with vinaigrette

This classic dish is so delicious it returns to our menu every year. Take extra care not to overcook the asparagus. White asparagus takes longer to cook than its green cousin, and thinner stalks should go into the pan slightly later than the thick ones.

Serves 8–10

2 bunches of white asparagus
1–2 bunches of green asparagus

Vinaigrette
3 large organic eggs, hardboiled
100 g (3 ½ oz) capers
1 large red onion
3 tsp olive oil
1 tsp white balsamic vinegar
½ tsp herb salt
2 tbsp roughly chopped parsley

Serves 40 children

6 bunches of white asparagus
8 bunches of green asparagus

Vinaigrette
15 large organic eggs, hardboiled
200 g (7 oz) capers
5 large red onions
200 ml (⅞ cup) olive oil
100 ml (½ cup) white balsamic vinegar
2 tsp herb salt
1 bunch of roughly chopped parsley

1. Peel and chop the eggs, chop the capers and onions, then mix together.
2. Mix a dressing of oil and vinegar and add salt and pepper to taste. Stir the dressing into the eggs and add the parsley.
3. Break off the woody ends of the green asparagus. Peel the white asparagus and cut the ends off (save all the ends for use in a vegetable stock).
4. Cook the green and white asparagus separately in plenty of lightly salted water. Leave the white to boil for around 5 minutes and the green for around 3 minutes.
5. Serve the asparagus immediately with a large spoonful of vinaigrette drizzled over each portion and a slice of bread. Yum!

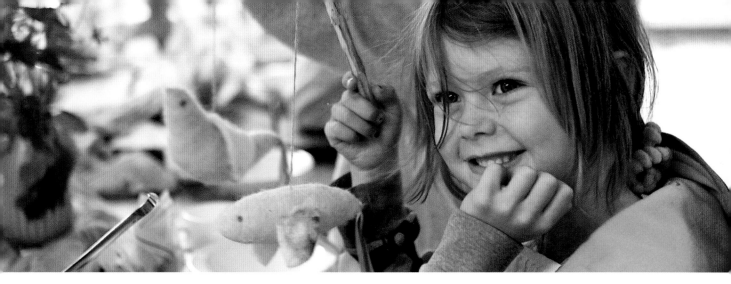

Asparagus pâté

All Danish nurseries have sandwich day once a week. This pâté is ideal for sandwiches as it can be made from leftovers and it is much cheaper and tastier than a lot of ready-made products.

Serves 8–10

1 bunch of green asparagus
4 organic eggs
5 tbsp dry black quinoa (or approx 170g leftover boiled rice)
150 g (5 ¼ oz) Öland wheat flour or spelt flour
200 ml (⅞ cup) herbal tea
1 tsp herb salt
freshly ground black pepper
1 onion, chopped

Serves 40 children

5 bunches of green asparagus
10 organic eggs
350 dl (250g) dry black quinoa (or approx. 750g leftover boiled rice)
420 g (15 oz) Öland wheat flour or spelt flour
600 ml (1¼ US pints) herbal tea
2 tsp herb salt
freshly ground black pepper
4 onions, chopped

1. Break off the lower ends of the asparagus and save them for use in a vegetable stock. Rinse the spears thoroughly under the cold tap and cut them into 2.5 cm (1 in) wide pieces.
2. Mix all the other ingredients in a large bowl and add the onions and asparagus.
3. Bake the pâté in a greased cake tin (25 cm/10 in diameter) at 180°C (350°F) for 20–30 minutes. Serve with salad and rye bread.

Spring tartlets

You will need to buy ready-made tartlet cases for this delicious springtime filling.

Serves a family of 4

1 bunch of green asparagus
½ bunch of white asparagus

Pesto
300 g (10 ½ oz) freshly picked ground elder (or another spring leaf)
200 g (7 oz) fresh parsley or spinach
1 tsp herb salt
150 g (5 ¼ oz) almonds
200 ml (⅞ cup) quality olive oil
zest of 1 organic lemon
2 tsp lemon juice
a handful of new beech leaves to garnish (optional)

Serves 40 children

10 bunches of green asparagus
5 bunches of white asparagus

Pesto
1 kg (2 lb 3 oz) freshly picked ground elder
500 g (1 lb 2 oz) fresh parsley
500 g (1 lb 2 oz) spinach
herb salt to taste
500 g (1 lb 2 oz) almonds
900 ml (2 US pints) quality olive oil
zest of 8 organic lemons
150 ml (⅔ cup) lemon juice
a few handfuls of new beech leaves to garnish (optional)

1. Break off the bottom ends of the asparagus and save them for use in a vegetable stock. Boil the green asparagus spears briefly in lightly salted water, then cut them into smaller pieces.
2. Peel the white asparagus and break off the ends (save them for use in a vegetable stock). Boil them in lightly salted water. Note that they take longer to cook than the green kind. Prick them with a sharp knife to see when they're done.
3. Put all the pesto ingredients, except for the lemon juice, in a blender and blend into a smooth paste. Finally add lemon juice to taste and possibly a pinch of salt and pepper.
4. Fold the asparagus into the pesto.
5. Warm up the tartlet cases, fill and serve immediately. Garnish with beech leaves.

As an alternative to ready-made tartlet cases, you could make your own puff pastry. It takes some time but the reward is an absolutely divine treat.

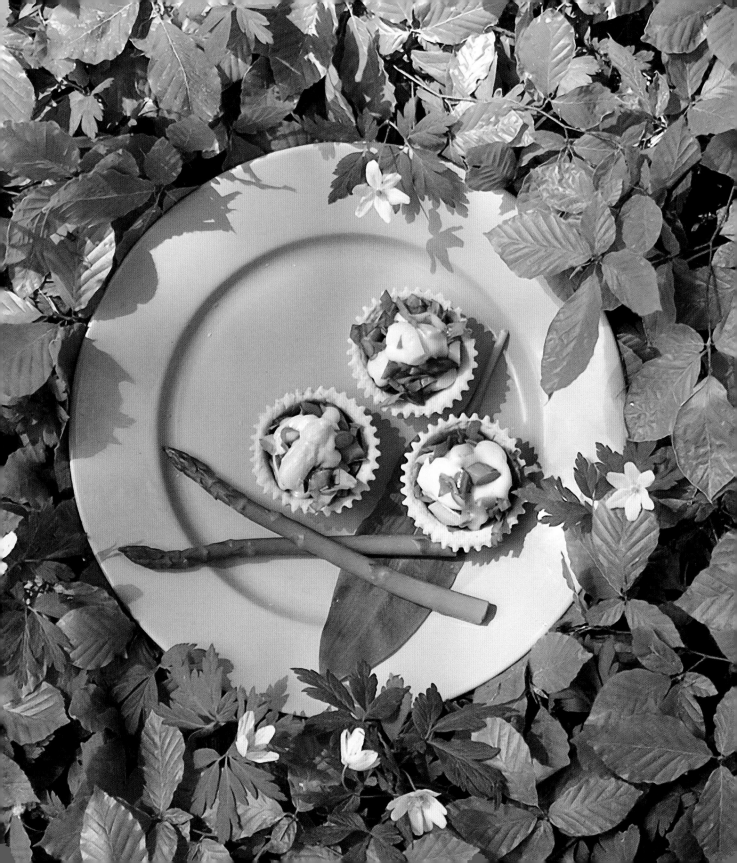

Spinach roulade with mashed carrots

By using amaranth seed flour instead of plain flour, you can make your spinach roulades suitable for people with a gluten allergy. Use any seasonal vegetables for your filling to add variety.

Serves 8–10
250 g (9 oz) blanched spinach
2 organic egg whites
¼ tsp grated nutmeg
½ tsp herb salt
freshly ground black pepper
1 tbsp amaranth seed flour or plain flour

Mashed carrots
500 g (1 lb 2 oz) peeled carrots
500 ml (1 US pint) water
1 tsp herb salt
2 tbsp quality oil

Serves 40 children
1 kg (2 lb 3 oz) blanched spinach
7–8 organic egg whites
1 tsp grated nutmeg
3 tsp herb salt
freshly ground black pepper
4 tbsp amaranth seed flour or plain flour

Mashed carrots
2 kg (4 lb 7 oz) peeled carrots
700 ml (1½ US pints) water
1 tsp herb salt
100 ml (½ cup) quality oil

1. Blanch the spinach in boiling water for about 10 seconds before immediately rinsing in ice-cold water. Chop the blanched spinach finely.
2. Stir the egg whites into the spinach and add the grated nutmeg, salt, pepper and flour.
3. Bake the spinach sheets as you would the layers of a sandwich (layer) cake: spread a thin layer of spinach mixture on a tin lined with greaseproof paper and bake for around 15–20 minutes at 180°C (350°F).
4. Boil the carrots for the filling until completely soft. Drain before puréeing with oil and salt.
5. Spread the purée thinly on the baked spinach sheets. Roll up the roulade carefully and store in the fridge until needed.
6. Slice the roulade finely with a sharp knife and serve as a sandwich filler or garnish.

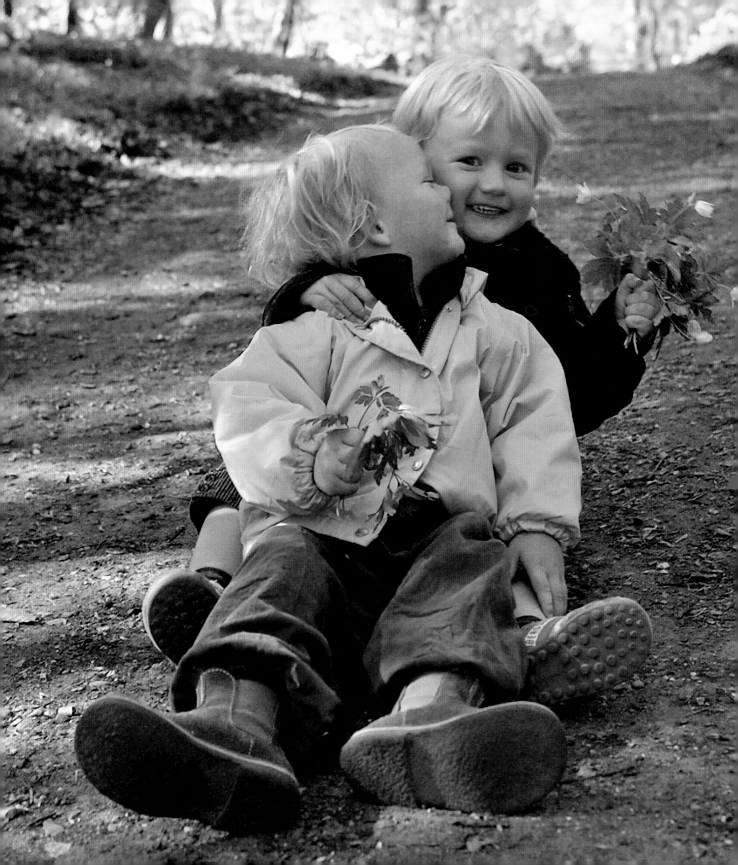

Crispbread

You can use leftovers such as boiled rice or porridge here instead of buckwheat. If you do, make sure you reduce the amount of water to 50 ml (¼ cup).

Makes 15–20 crispbreads
45 g (1 ½ oz) buckwheat flakes
70 g (2 ½ oz) sesame seeds
65 g (2 ⅓ oz) sunflower seeds
130 g (4 ½ oz) plain or spelt flour
130 g (4 ½ oz) graham or spelt flour
1 tsp salt
100 ml (½ cup) thistle oil
approx. 150 ml (⅔ cup) water or cold herbal tea

1. Mix the dry ingredients and knead the dough smooth with oil and water.
2. Roll the dough out thinly onto greaseproof paper and cut it into shapes with a pizza cutter or scissors.
3. Bake the bread at 200°C (400°F) for around 20 minutes.
4. You can store the bread for up to two weeks in a tin.

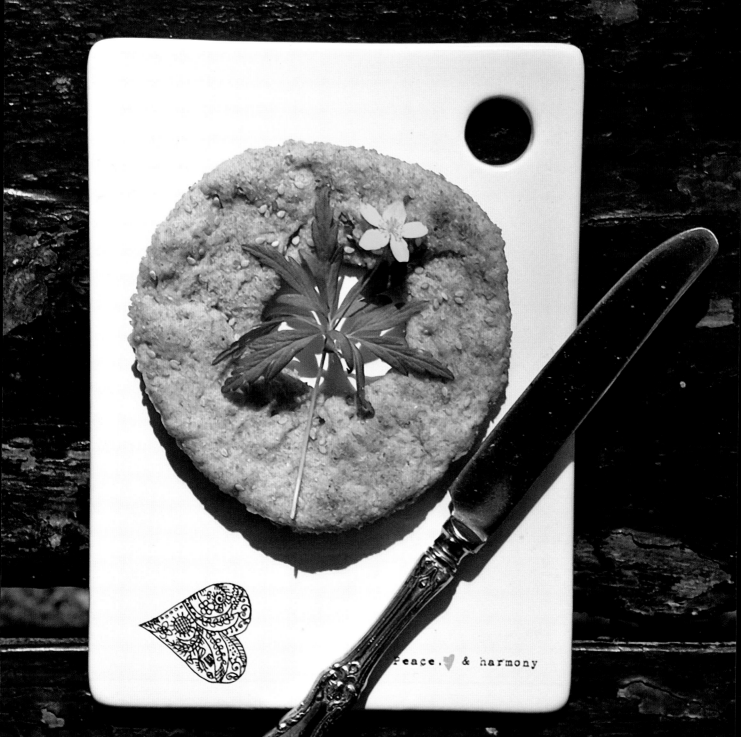

peace, 💙 & harmony

Carrot soup

The flavour of this soup is divine and its colour golden. Orange peel adds an extra dimension to the carrots and the bowls will always be wiped clean. It can be enjoyed hot or ice cold on a warm summer's day.

Serves a family of 4
500 g (1 lb 2 oz) carrots
450 g (1 lb) potatoes
150 g (5 ¼ oz) celeriac
2 onions
1 tsp oil
water
1 can of organic coconut milk
juice and zest of 1 organic orange
1 pinch of freshly grated ginger
1 clove of garlic
1 tsp white balsamic vinegar
1 tsp agave syrup
½ tsp cayenne pepper
herb salt
freshly ground black pepper

Serves 40 children
5 kg (11 lb) carrots
3 kg (6 lb 10 oz) potatoes
1 kg (2lb 3 oz) celeriac
500 g (1 lb 2 oz) onions
2 tbsp oil
water
5 cans of organic coconut milk
juice and zest of 2 organic oranges
2 tsp freshly grated ginger
3 cloves of garlic
5 tsp white balsamic vinegar
3 tsp agave syrup
1–2 tsp cayenne pepper
herb salt
freshly ground black pepper

1. Peel the carrots, potatoes, celeriac and onions, dice them roughly, and sauté in oil in a heavy pan.
2. Add water until the vegetables are almost covered, then add the coconut milk and stir in the orange juice, orange zest, ginger and garlic.
3. When the vegetables have softened, blend and add the vinegar, agave syrup, cayenne and salt and pepper to taste.
4. You can garnish the soup with marinated pearl barley or rye bread croutons.

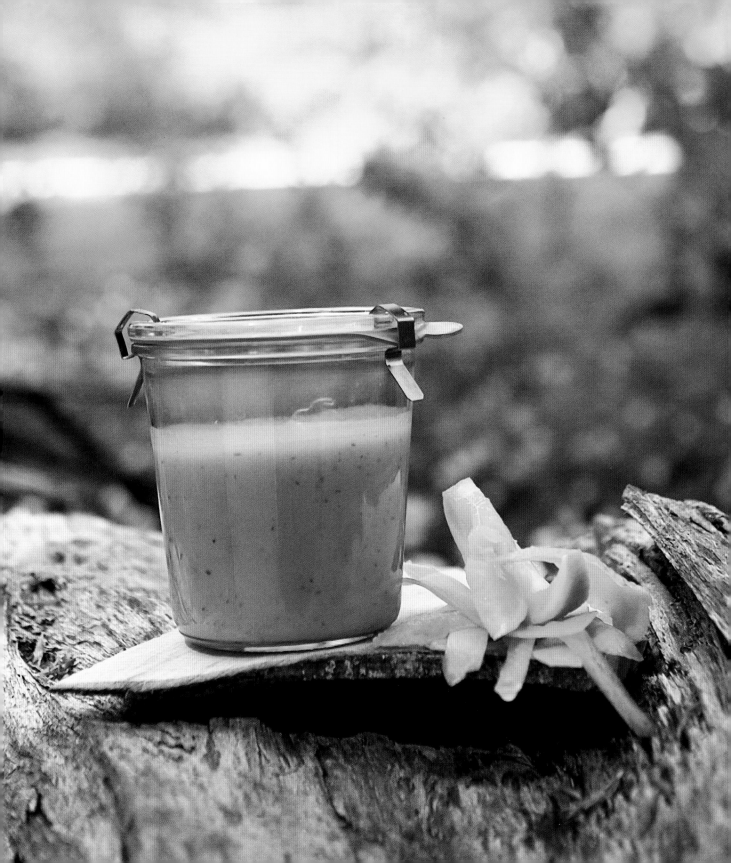

Carrot curry

This curry is very popular with all our children because the carrots taste sweet and familiar. The flavour of new carrots is incredible.

Serves a family of 4
1.5 kg (3 lb 5 oz) carrots
2 onions
1 tbsp coriander seeds
5 cardamom pods
1 tsp pink peppercorns
1 tsp allspice
2 mild red chillies
4 cloves of garlic
2–3 limes
40 g (1½ oz) fresh ginger
2 tbsp thistle oil
500 ml (1 US pint) organic coconut milk
1 tsp herb salt

Serves 40 children
7 kg (15 lb 7 oz) carrots
10 onions
4 tbsp coriander seeds
15 cardamom pods
4 tsp pink peppercorns
4 tsp allspice
4 mild red chillies
12 cloves of garlic
9 limes
120 g (4¼ oz) fresh ginger
200 ml (1 cup) thistle oil
2.5 l (5¼ US pints) organic coconut milk
4 tsp herb salt

1. Peel the carrots and cut them into 2.5 cm (1 in) wide slices. Chop the onions.
2. Grind the coriander seeds, cardamom seeds (the little black seeds inside the pods), pink peppercorns, allspice, chillies and garlic into a thick paste in a mortar.
3. Mix the juice from the limes with the freshly grated ginger.
4. Sauté the carrots and onions in the oil in a pan for at least 15 minutes.
5. Add the spice paste and let it fry over a high heat for around 10 seconds.
6. Pour in the lime juice and coconut milk. Leave to simmer until creamy.
7. Add salt to taste, and serve the curry with rice or something similar.

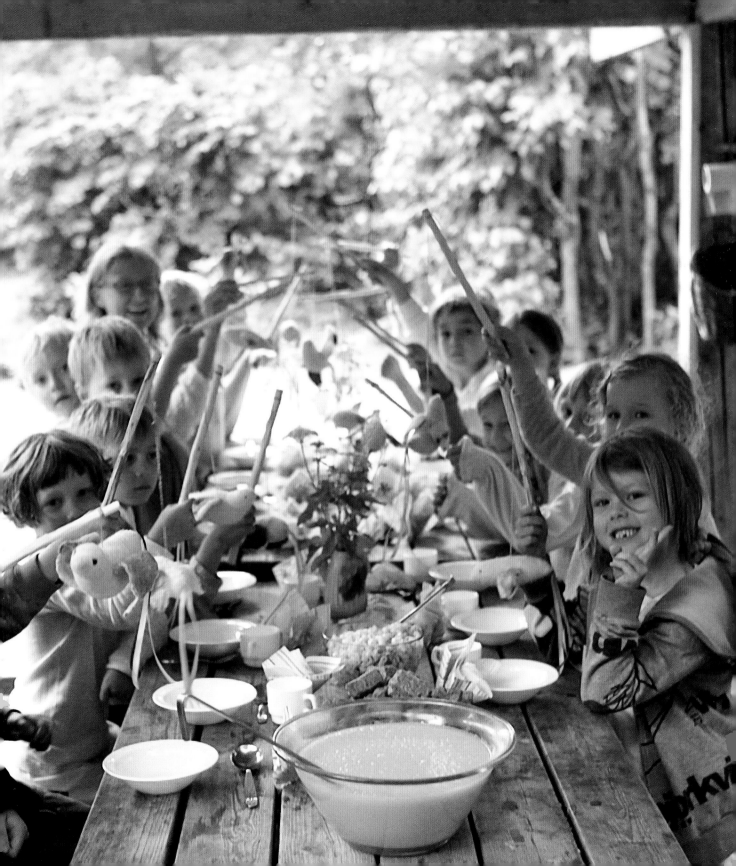

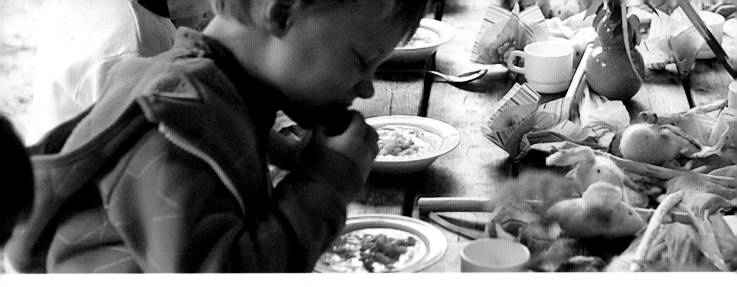

Carrots with satay sauce

You can serve satay sauce with almost any type of vegetable or as a dip.

Serves a family of 4
1 kg (2 lb 3 oz) carrots

Satay sauce
250 g (9 oz) peanut butter
juice of 1 organic lemon
½ tsp cayenne pepper
1 tsp herb salt
200–300 ml (1–1 ¼ cups) boiling water from
  the carrots

Serves 40 children
7 kg (15 lb 7 oz) carrots

Satay sauce
680 g (1 lb 8 oz) peanut butter
juice of 5 organic lemons
3 tsp cayenne pepper
4 tsp herb salt
800–1000 ml (1 ⅔–2 US pints) water from the
  boiled carrots

1. Peel the carrots and cut them into 5 cm (2 in) thick pieces.
2. Boil them in lightly salted water until soft (around 7–10 minutes). Remember to set aside some of the water for the satay sauce.
3. Mix all the ingredients for the satay sauce and slowly stir in the water, until the sauce is a good consistency.
4. Fold in the carrots and serve.

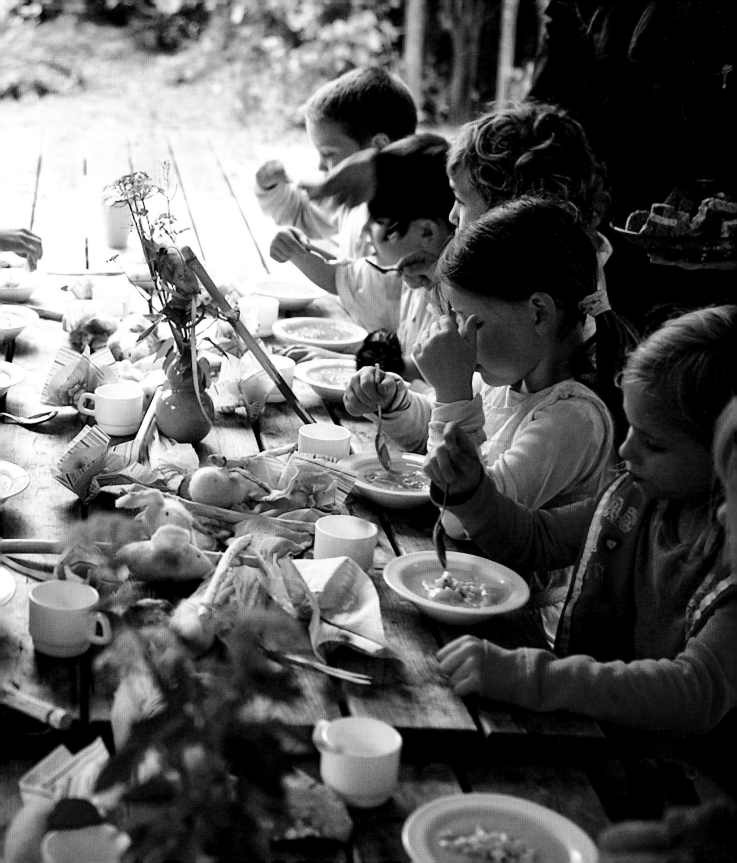

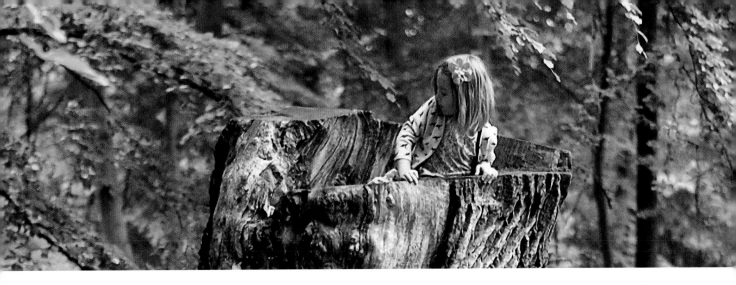

Spinach pesto

This is full of selenium and iron.

Serves 8	Serves 40 children
500 g (1 lb 2 oz) fresh spinach	2.5 kg (5 lb 8 oz) fresh spinach
250 g (9 oz) Brazil nuts	1 kg (2 lb 3 oz) Brazil nuts
100 g (3 ½ oz) Parmesan cheese	500 g (1 lb 2 oz) Parmesan cheese
1 tbsp capers	4–5 tbsp capers
100–200 ml (½–1 small cup) olive oil	1 l (2 US pints) olive oil
1–2 cloves of garlic	6–7 cloves of garlic
1 tsp herb salt	4 tsp herb salt

1. Wash the spinach very thoroughly, changing the water at least 3 times, or even better, 7!
2. Put all the ingredients in a blender, or use a handheld mixer, and blend to your desired consistency.
3. Store the pesto in a clean glass jar. It can be used for up to a week.
4. Serve with wholegrain pasta. Use 3.2 kg (7 lb) dry pasta for 40 children.

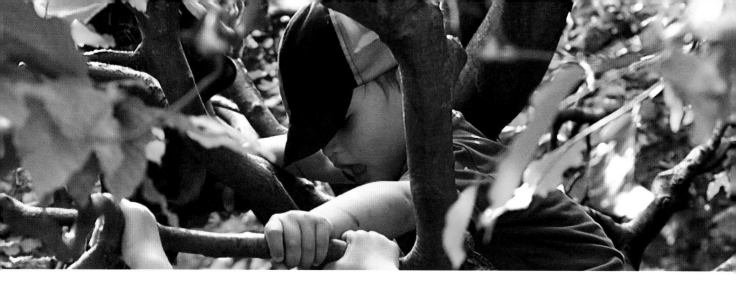

Spinach lasagne

This a true vegetarian classic, for good reason. it tastes great and the children love it.

Serves a family of 4
500 g (1 lb 2 oz) ricotta cheese
1 can of chopped tomatoes
1 tsp herb salt
1 tsp nutmeg and crushed fennel seeds
a splash of organic lemon juice
1 kg (2 lb 3 oz) blanched spinach
1 pack of fresh lasagne sheets
100 g (3 ½ oz) Parmesan cheese

Serves 40 children
3 kg (6 lb 10 oz) ricotta cheese
5 cans of chopped tomatoes
5 tsp herb salt
3 tsp nutmeg and crushed fennel seeds
juice of 2 organic lemons
5 kg (11 lb) blanched spinach
5 packs of fresh lasagne sheets
1 kg (2 lb 3 oz) Parmesan cheese

1. Mix together the ricotta, tomatoes, salt, nutmeg, fennel and lemon juice.
2. Squeeze the liquid out of the blanched spinach, chop it roughly and add it to the rest of the filling (see p. 40 on how to blanch spinach).
3. Assemble the lasagne in a buttered dish. Start and end with a layer of filling, and top with grated Parmesan.
4. Cook the lasagne for 30 minutes at 200°C (400°F).

Spring rolls

Children love eating these with their fingers. Spring roll sheets can be found in Asian supermarkets, but unfortunately there are not usually organic versions.

Makes 10 rolls

1 sweetheart cabbage
5–6 spring onions
2 large carrots
2 tbsp quality oil
spring roll sheets (available in Asian
   supermarkets or get wholegrain sheets
   from www.levadelsrollitos.com)
1 organic egg white
200 ml (⅞ cup) corn or sunflower oil for
   deep-frying
1 tbsp water

1. Chop the cabbage and spring onions finely. Peel and grate the carrots.
2. Sauté the vegetables lightly in oil in a frying pan without letting them brown.
3. Beat the egg white and water.
4. Distribute the spring roll sheets across a large table and place a dollop of filling in the middle of each sheet, fold the ends in and roll into a cigar shape. Brush the edges with the egg mix to seal.
5. Heat the oil in a pan, but don't let it get too hot. Deep-fry the spring rolls and leave them to drain on a sheet of kitchen roll.
6. Serve with tamari or soy sauce, steamed vegetables and boiled rice.

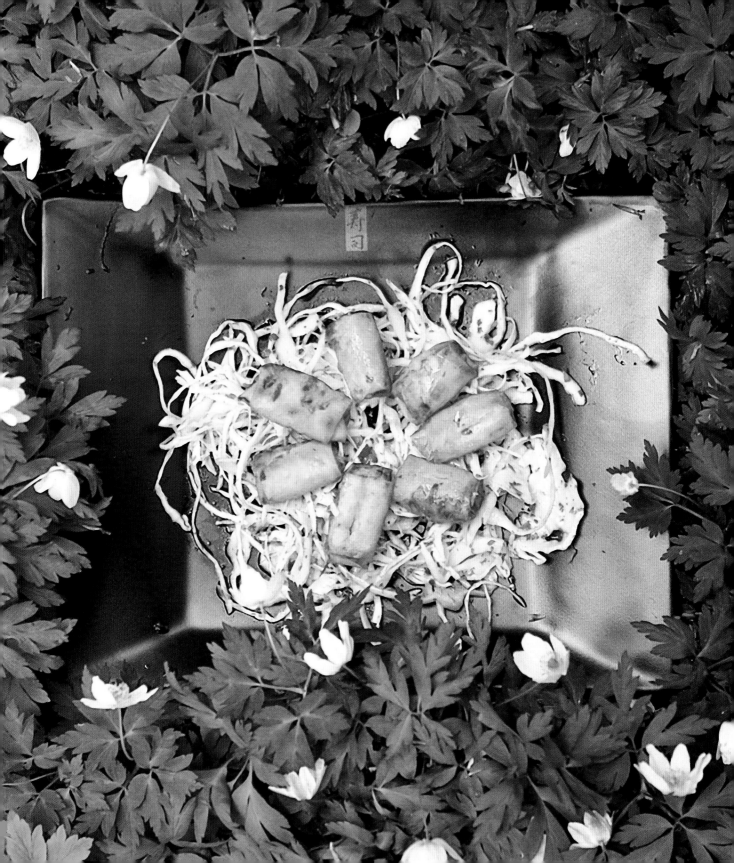

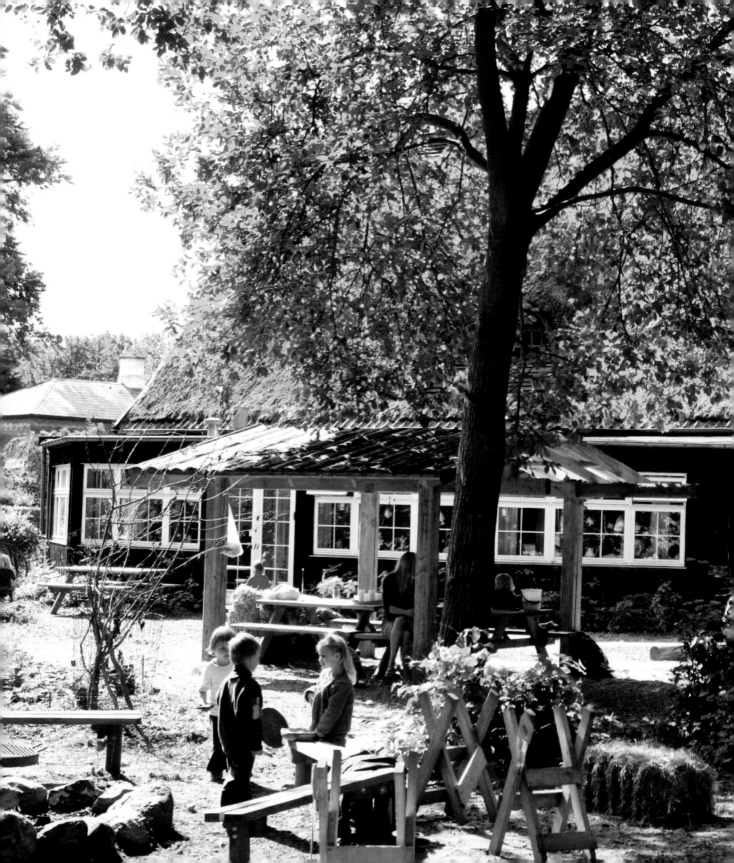

Summer

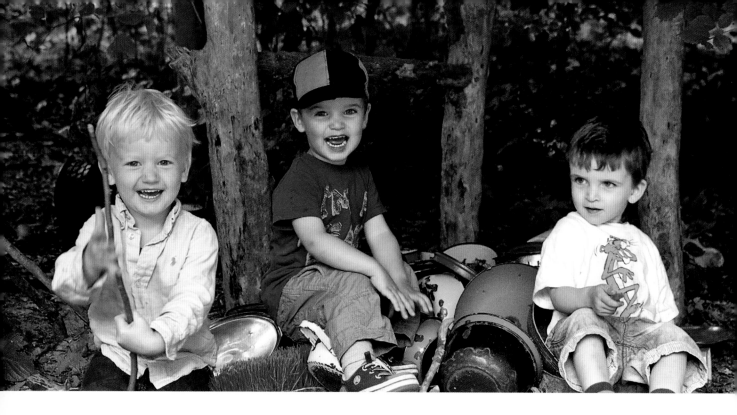

Nights are short; days are long. The sun rises early and the northern hemisphere turns towards the light. The temperature rises, clothes are shed and we wiggle our bare toes in our sandals, which have returned from their exile at the back of the wardrobe. The world grows lighter, everything hums with life and everywhere you look things are crawling, growing. The forest is dense and lush and full of wonderful shade; the sea is blue as though someone's painted it, and the grass becomes a plush rug. In other words: it's summer!

Summer means outdoor activities, and the children instinctively seek out the shade under the trees, because if there's one thing children don't like, it's being in direct sunlight. Our meals are influenced by the coming of summer too; most families unwind, the rhythm of family life slows

down and the line between playing outdoors and mealtimes gets blurred.

Summer fruits and vegetables have a high water content, which is ideal as we need plenty of water to stay hydrated in the summer heat. It's easy to eat a varied diet and not get stuck with the same old dishes during the summer, because there are always wonderful fresh vegetables in our shops and gardens – for those of us lucky enough to have access to one. The summer crops seem to be trying to outgrow nature's own wild plants and grasses; everything is lush and inviting. There's no need to huddle over the hob for hours like in wintertime because crisp summer salads almost make themselves.

In summer it's easy to involve children in helping with food preparation, not least because a lot of the cooking can be done outdoors.

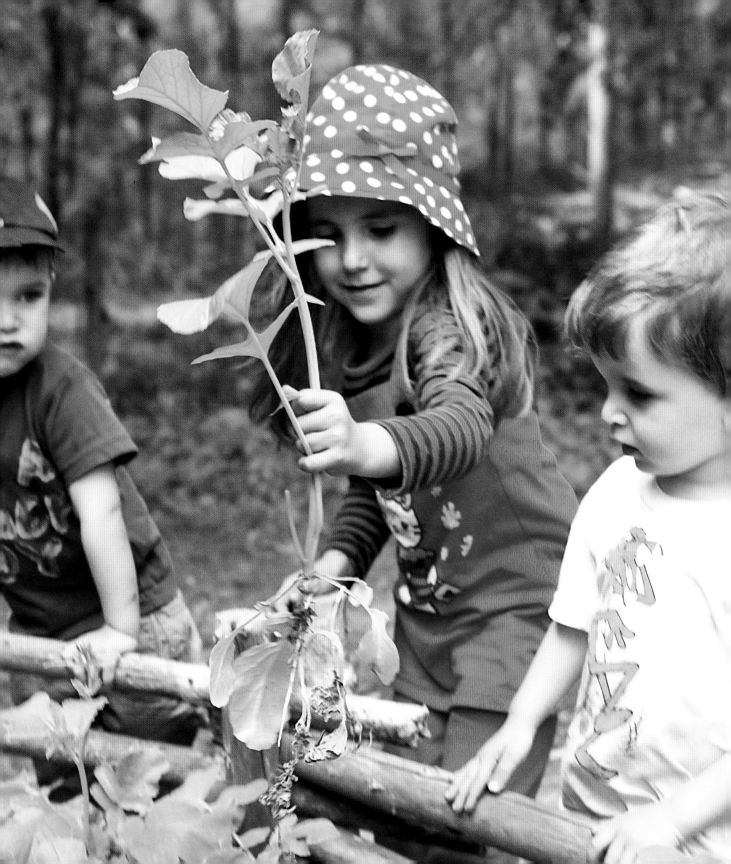

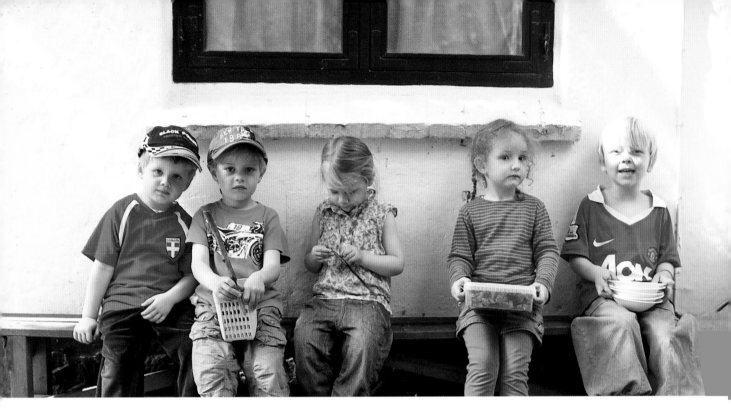

The range of available vegetables is extensive and colourful and packed with different flavours. It's easy to let children explore while you scrub, peel and chop vegetables, berries, fruits or herbs. In fact, herbs deserve a chapter all to themselves; they are so much more than just 'green garnish' and they can be the magic ingredients that really make a salad.

Pick-your-own fruit and berries

It's a sure sign that summer is here when the bushes are heavy with berries. Sweet berries, sour berries, blackberries, bitter berries – and first and foremost strawberries! The berries in Northern Europe are generally very flavoursome because it takes them longer to ripen up here. Therefore,

it might be worthwhile waiting for local berries instead of buying the ones from the south, which appear in the shops much earlier in the year.

After the strawberries come the raspberries, then the currants and blackberries, which last into early autumn. The first apples appear in August, with rosehips hard on their heels. Most children love picking their own berries, armed with their own basket.

The kitchen garden

At Bonsai we have planted a kitchen garden near the house and it has been life affirming to see how happy the children are to join in with gardening, helping out with weeding and watering. The first things to sprout are radishes, which aren't the

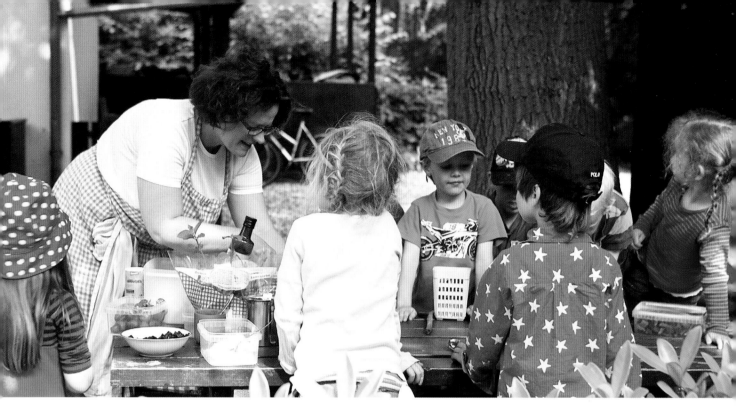

most popular vegetable with children. But when they have grown them and pulled them out of the ground themselves, it's a different story; almost all children will happily eat their own, freshly harvested radishes.

It's a good idea to keep a small herb garden, maybe just in a window box, where plants can sprout throughout the summer. It requires some time and effort, of course, but it's extremely gratifying and children enjoy it; growing things with your children is a lovely thing to do.

Plan your crops so that there will be something to harvest most of the time, because if there's a long period with nothing happening, children tend to lose interest. We have planted potatoes, lettuce and herbs, but you can ask for advice at your garden centre or consult a sowing calendar.

How to churn butter

Fill a clean jar with a lid to the quarter mark with double cream. Screw the lid on tight and let the children shake the jar. After about five minutes there will be a small, yellow blob of butter in the middle. Keep shaking and suddenly all the cream will turn into delicious, home-churned butter, which tastes particularly good on freshly baked bread, because you made it yourselves! The butter can be stored in the fridge for up to a week.

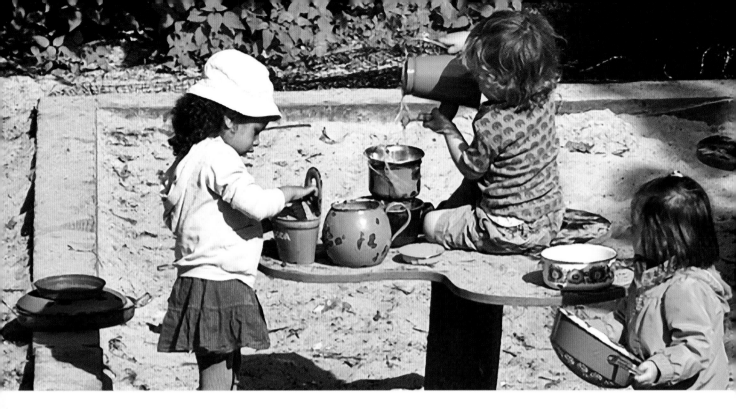

Harvest festival

The harvest season begins at the end of summer. Nature is brimming with fruit and vegetables and everything is bursting with abundance. After the summer holidays we start preparing for the harvest festival.

Visit a farm

Most small farms welcome visitors, and a farm visit can be a great thing to do with children, both because they enjoy it and because they learn a lot. At Bonsai we go on an annual trip to see farmer Henrik down on Kragebjerg farm. Henrik grows crops and keeps animals and he follows biodynamic principles. This means, for example, that the children can pull carrots out of the ground, wipe off the dirt on their trousers and bite straight into them, because no chemicals have been used. And they are always happy to do just that! Farmer Henrik also shows them how grain was harvested in the past with a scythe, and we help him gather the grain into sheaves, which we can then take home for our kindergarten harvest festival.

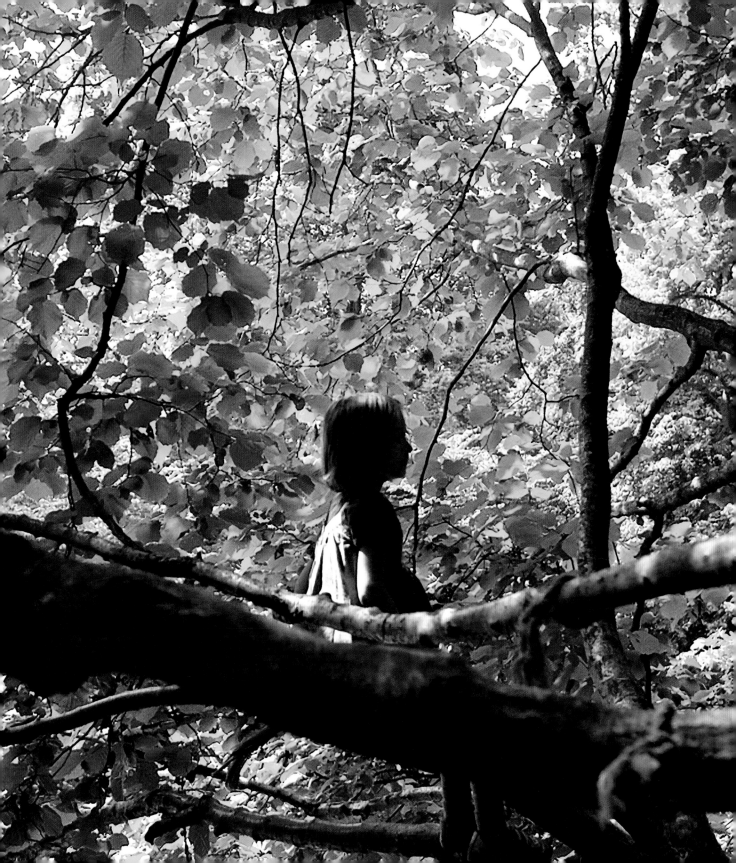

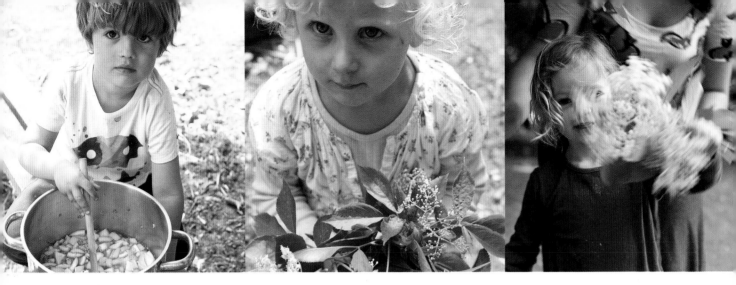

Elderflower cordial

This is a summer classic. Take your children to pick elderflowers. They will love picking the flowers and drinking the squash that they helped to make.

Serves 40 children
1 ½ organic lemons
1 kg (2 lb 3 oz) sugar
1 l (2 US pints) water
25 large elderflower heads

1. Slice the lemons and put them in a large pan with the sugar.
2. Add water and bring to the boil.
3. Put the flowers in large bowl and pour over the hot liquid. Cover and leave in a cool place for 3 days.
4. Strain the cordial through a coffee filter and bottle it.
5. Serve 1 part cordial to 3 parts water.

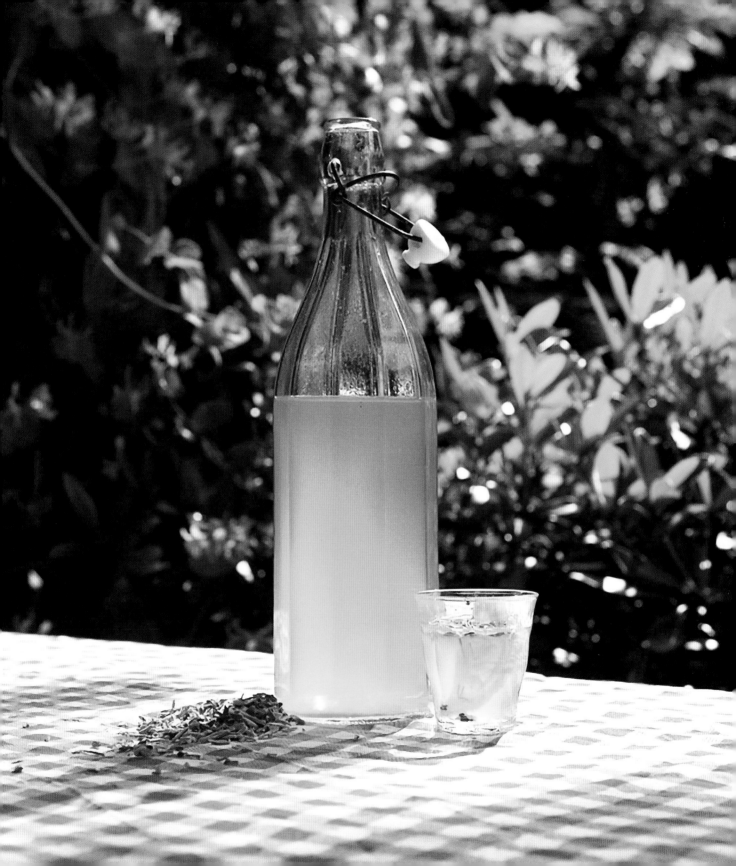

Tomato ketchup

My children love ketchup and for a while they ate it with everything, which made me quite keen to find an alternative. I tried various recipes, pouring it into old ketchup bottles to make the substitute easier to accept. But they didn't buy it! Instead we tried tasting the ketchup together, and I came up with adding apricots (really ripe ones) in summer and apples in winter. It now goes down exceedingly well with both the children and the adults.

Makes 700 ml (1 ½ US pints) of ketchup

600 g (1 lb 5 oz) fresh apricots or
  500 g (1 lb 2 oz) apple sauce (in autumn/
  winter)
500 g (1 lb 2 oz) ripe tomatoes
500 g (1 lb 2 oz) demerara sugar
2–3 tbsp tomato purée
1 tsp cayenne pepper
3 tbsp lemon juice
3 tbsp white balsamic vinegar
1–2 tsp herb salt

1. Blanch the apricots, peel them and remove the stalks.
2. Remove the stalks from the tomatoes, blanch and peel them and remove the seeds.
3. Blend the apricots and tomatoes and pour the mix into a heavy pan.
4. Add the sugar and tomato purée, and let the ketchup simmer for 30–40 minutes.
5. Add the lemon juice, vinegar, cayenne and herb salt to taste.
6. Let the ketchup cool before bottling it.

To make sure the bottles are thoroughly clean, wash them in the dishwasher and only take them out when you are ready to bottle the ketchup. Then seal the bottles carefully and boil them in water for a few minutes.

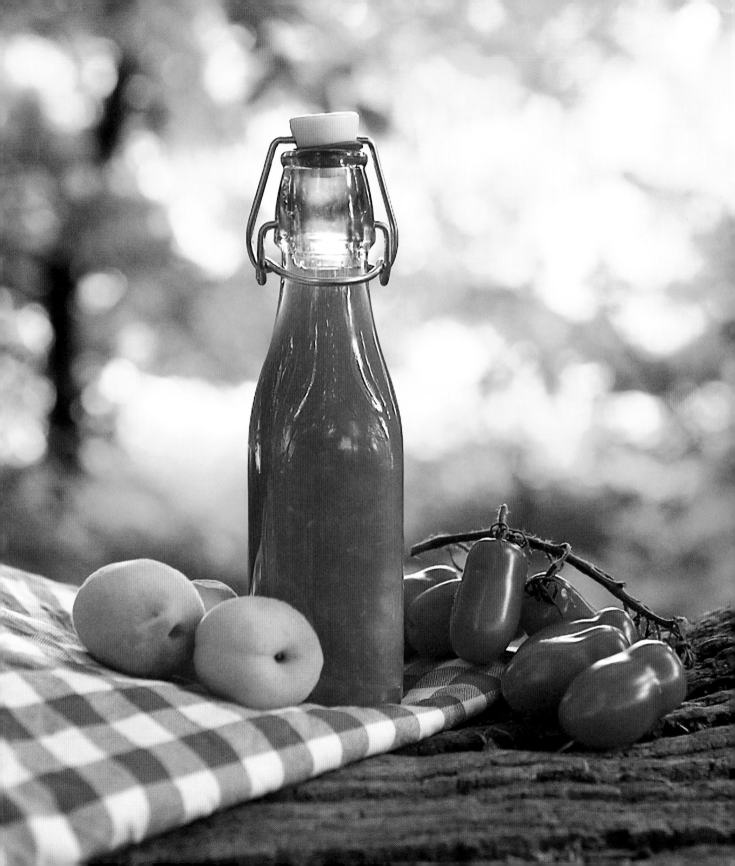

Tomato and millet tabbouleh

Millet is very rich in selenium, which is particularly important in a vegetarian diet. Whole millet grains can be soaked in water overnight to reduce the cooking time.

Serves a family of 4
250 g (9 oz) millet grains
1 cucumber
4–5 ripe tomatoes
½ bunch of parsley

Dressing
1–2 cloves of garlic
3 tbsp olive oil
1 tbsp white balsamic vinegar
1 tsp herb salt

Serves 40 children
2 kg (4 lb 7 oz) millet grains
8 large cucumbers
16 ripe tomatoes
2 bunches of parsley

Dressing
4–5 cloves of garlic
12 tbsp olive oil
5 tbsp white balsamic vinegar
4 tsp herb salt

1. Rinse the millet and boil it for at least 30 minutes. Soaking the millet overnight will reduce the cooking time.
2. Dice the cucumbers and tomatoes, and finely chop the parsley. You might consider letting the children cut the tomatoes using a small bread knife.
3. Peel and chop the garlic finely; you can adjust the amount of garlic to your own taste.
4. Mix a dressing of oil, vinegar and salt, then add the garlic.
5. Mix all the ingredients for the tabbouleh, toss with the dressing and let it rest for a while.
6. Serve as a side dish, starter or light lunch with a nice hunk of bread.

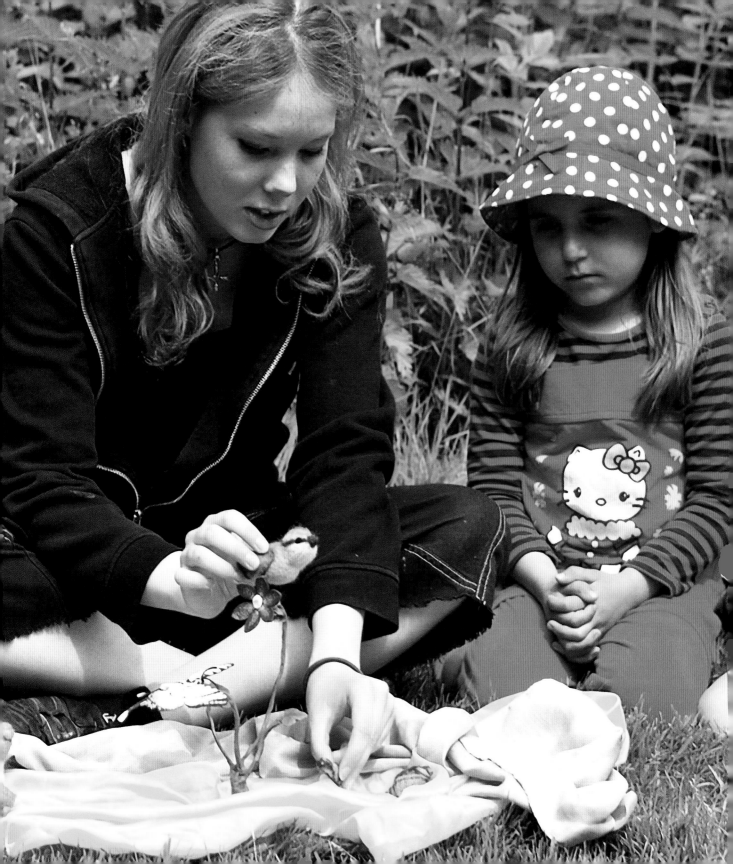

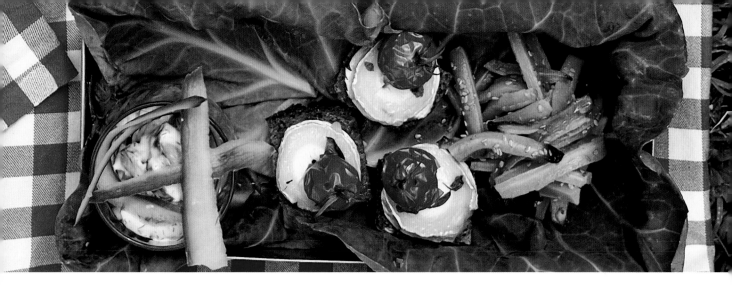

Tomato crostini

Crostini are a firm summer favourite with Italians. They're a wonderful way of using up leftovers. The melted cheese on top is optional.

Serves a family of 4
8 slices of day-old bread
1 clove of garlic
3 tbsp olive oil
8 slices of goat's or Emmental cheese
8–10 cherry tomatoes
1 pinch of herb salt
10 basil leaves

Serves 40 children
60 slices of day-old bread
4 cloves of garlic
300 ml (1¼ cups) olive oil
1 kg (2 lb 3 oz) goat's or Emmental cheese
4 punnets of cherry tomatoes
2 tsp herb salt
1 bunch of basil leaves

1. Rub the bread slices with the garlic cloves and sprinkle them with oil.
2. Place the bread on greaseproof paper and put 1 slice of goat's cheese, 1 basil leaf and 1 thinly sliced cherry tomato on each slice. If you're using Emmental cheese, you might prefer to grate it on top.
3. Bake the crostini in the oven for 15 minutes at 180°C (350°F) and serve as a starter or a snack.

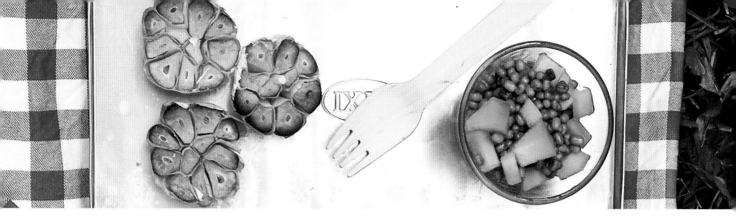

Mung bean and melon salad

Serves a family of 4
250 g (9 oz) mung beans
1 cantaloupe melon
pea shoots (optional)

Dressing
2 tbsp olive oil
1 tsp lemon juice
1 tsp salt

Serves 40 children
2.5 kg (5 lb 8 oz) mung beans
5 cantaloupe melons
pea shoots (optional)

Dressing
300 ml (1¼ cups) olive oil
100 ml (½ cup) lemon juice
2 tsp salt

1. Boil the mung beans in lightly salted water for 25 minutes, until they're soft. Mung beans don't require pre-soaking and they have a delicious flavour, similar to peas.
2. Peel the melon and remove the seeds. Chop the flesh into small pieces.
3. Mix a dressing of oil, lemon juice and salt.
4. You can use pea shoots to garnish the dish and complement and lift the flavours.

Roasted garlic

It can be difficult to get through a kilo of garlic in kindergarten, which is the smallest order our suppliers deliver. A useful trick is to bake any leftover garlic. Roasting also makes the flavour milder, and it is delicious in dressings and pâtés. By infusing oil with roasted garlic you will always have flavour readily to hand.

Cut each bulb in half, and peel off the excess skin. Place the halves on greaseproof paper and brush them with oil and herb salt. Roast the garlic at 200°C (400°F) for around 25–30 minutes. The garlic can then be stored in the fridge in a plastic container for up to 2 days.

Potato pizza

I still remember the first time I tried potato pizza, at Café Victor during the last months of catering college. It was so delicious, but back then putting potato on pizza seemed much too Danish for an Italian dish – like when people used to fill French croissants with chicken salad in the eighties. Now, post fusion food, Nordic pizza seems likes a wonderful thing!

Serves a family of 4
10 g (⅓ oz) fresh yeast
500 ml (1 US pint) tepid water
approx. 1 kg (2 lb 3 oz) Öland wheat flour
2 tbsp oil
pinch of herb salt
3 tbsp bran

Topping
4–6 sliced new potatoes
50 g (1 ¾ oz / ½ jar) capers
2 tbsp oil for brushing

Serves 40 children
25 g (1 oz) fresh yeast
1.5 l (3 US pints) tepid water
approx. 3 kg (6 lb 10 oz) Öland wheat flour
100 ml (½ cup) oil
1 tbsp herb salt
60 g (2 oz) bran

Topping
2 kg (4 lb 7 oz) sliced new potatoes
200 g (7 oz/2 jars) capers
4 tbsp oil for brushing

1. Dissolve the yeast in the lukewarm water then add the flour little by little.
2. Add the oil, salt and bran to the dough.
3. Knead it thoroughly and leave it to prove in a cool place overnight.
4. Roll out the dough into several mini pizzas or 1 large pizza.
5. Clean the new potatoes and cut them into thin slices.
6. Arrange the potato slices on the pizza base and scatter with capers. Then brush with oil.
7. Bake the pizzas at 200°C (400°F). The baking time will depend on the size of the pizzas.

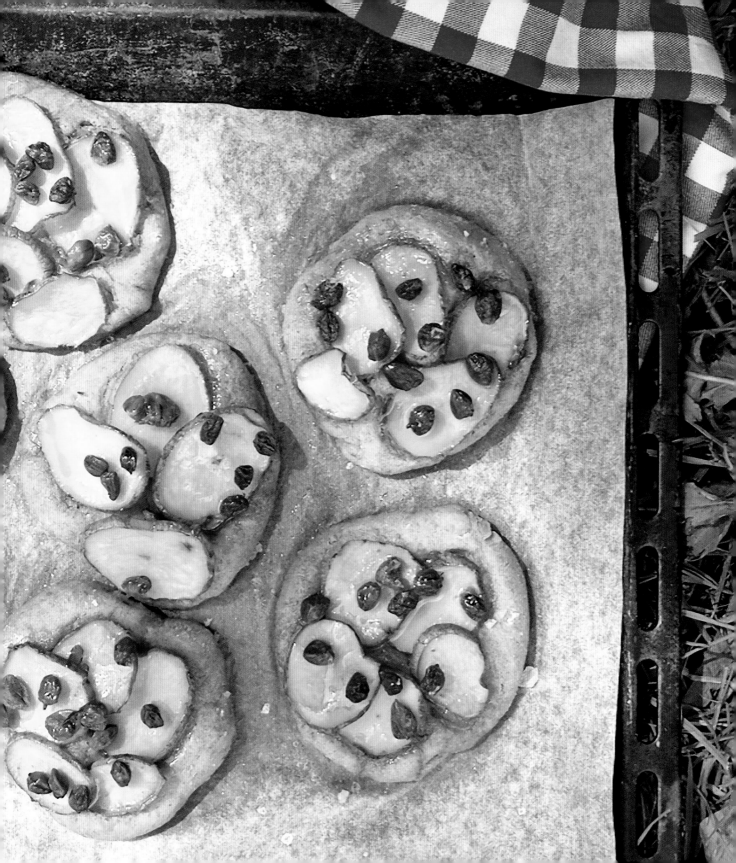

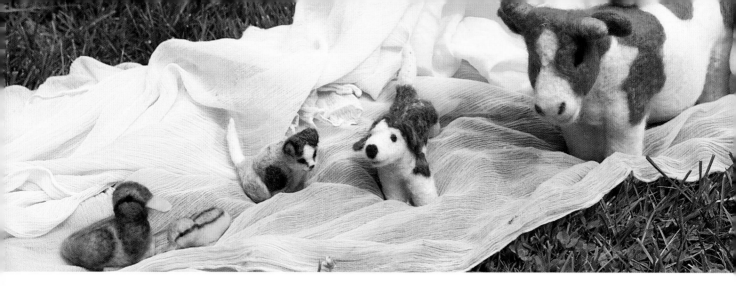

Warm potato salad

This old-fashioned potato salad is delicious, and always results in more empty plates than the more standard version made with mayonnaise.

Serves a family of 4
500 g (1 lb 2 oz) new potatoes
2 onions
100 ml (½ cup) thistle oil
2 tbsp cider vinegar
5 sprigs of dill
herb salt
freshly ground pepper
1 tbsp acacia honey
leafy green herbs (optional)

Serves 40 children
3 kg (6 lb 10 oz) new potatoes
7 onions
300 ml (1 ¼ cups) thistle oil
6 tbsp cider vinegar
1 bunch of dill
herb salt
freshly ground pepper
100 ml (½ cup) acacia honey
leafy green herbs (optional)

1. Scrub the potatoes well, boil them until soft then drain.
2. Chop the onions finely and fry lightly in oil.
3. Add the vinegar, honey, finely chopped dill and salt and pepper to taste.
4. Slice the potatoes and toss immediately with the dressing.
5. You could also add a variety of finely chopped, leafy herbs. Lovage is particularly good.

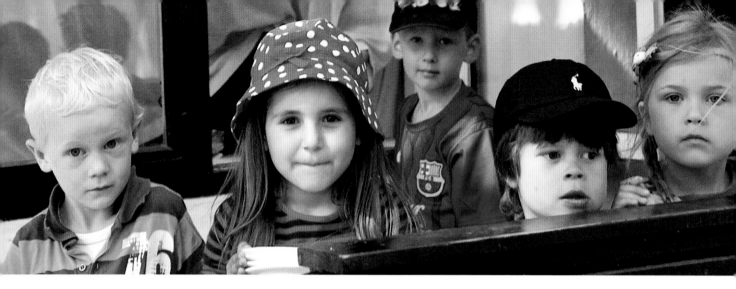

Potato balls

These meatless balls can be made using all kinds of vegetables and leftovers. Remember to adjust the amount of flour to make a good consistency.

Serves a family of 4
250 g (9 oz) new potatoes
1 onion
2 organic eggs
80 g (2 ¾ oz) cooked quinoa
125 g (4 ½ oz) spelt flour
1 tsp herb salt
green herbs
oil for frying

Serves 40 children
4 kg (8lb 13 oz) new potatoes
5 onions
10 organic eggs
300 g (10 ½ oz) cooked quinoa
500 g (1 lb 2 oz) spelt flour
3 tbsp herb salt
green herbs
oil for frying

1. Scrub the potatoes, peel the onion and grate both.
2. Stir in the eggs, quinoa, spelt flour and salt.
3. If you are using herbs, chop them and add them too.
4. Let the mash rest, covered, for 15 minutes in a cool place or the fridge.
5. Use a large teaspoon to shape balls the right size for the children, and fry in oil.

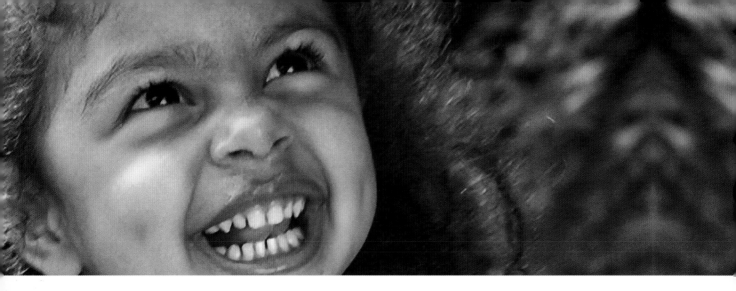

Easy strawberry ice lollies

This year we went strawberry picking and returned with several kilos of berries. So I invented this simple recipe, which was a huge hit. Make big batches as these lollies have a tendency to disappear very quickly!

Makes 12 lollies
1 l (2 US pints) organic natural yoghurt
1 punnet of strawberries
100 ml (½ cup) agave syrup
½ vanilla pod

1. Rinse and hull (remove the top of) the strawberries.
2. Add the agave syrup to the berries and purée.
3. Scrape the seeds out of the vanilla pod and stir them into the yoghurt along with the strawberry purée.
4. Fill small ice-lolly moulds with the mixture and freeze. Allow at least 10 hours freezing time before serving.

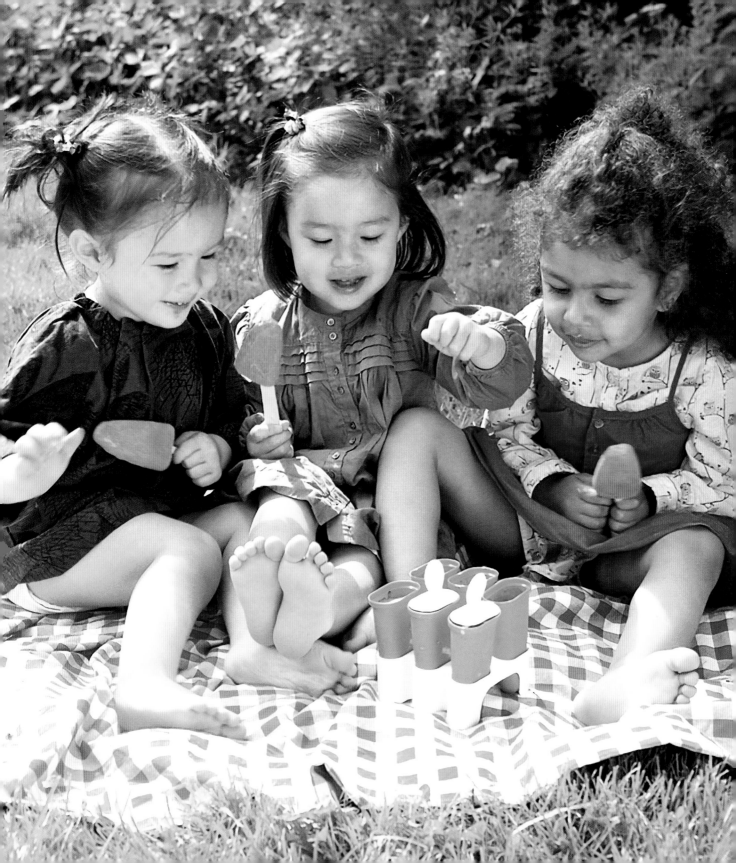

Kindergarten-style strawberry smoothie

This tofu smoothie, rich in protein, fibre and fat, is a truly great snack when accompanied with a piece of wholegrain bread.

Serves 40 children
2 l (4¼ US pints) rice milk
1.5 kg (3 lb 5 oz) strawberries
3 tbsp bran
2 tbsp thistle oil
250 g (9 oz) silken tofu

1. Prepare the ingredients and blend them until smooth.
2. Serve the smoothie in a small cup with a straw and a hunk of rye bread.

• •

Strawberry iced tea

This sweet iced tea with a hint of liquorice is refreshing and healthy. We often serve it in the summer, when it is particularly hot outside and the children need extra fluids. You could put strawberries in an ice-cube tray, add water, freeze and serve the iced tea with fun strawberry ice cubes.

Makes 2 litres (4 US pints)
1 l (2 US pints) water
2 tbsp sliced liquorice root
1 tbsp agave syrup
150 g (5 ¼ oz) strawberries
10–15 ice cubes

1. Bring the water to the boil and pour it over the liquorice root. Leave to steep for around 15 minutes.
2. Stir in the agave syrup and leave to cool.
3. Meanwhile, rinse and hull the strawberries and quarter them.
4. Serve the iced tea with strawberries and ice cubes.

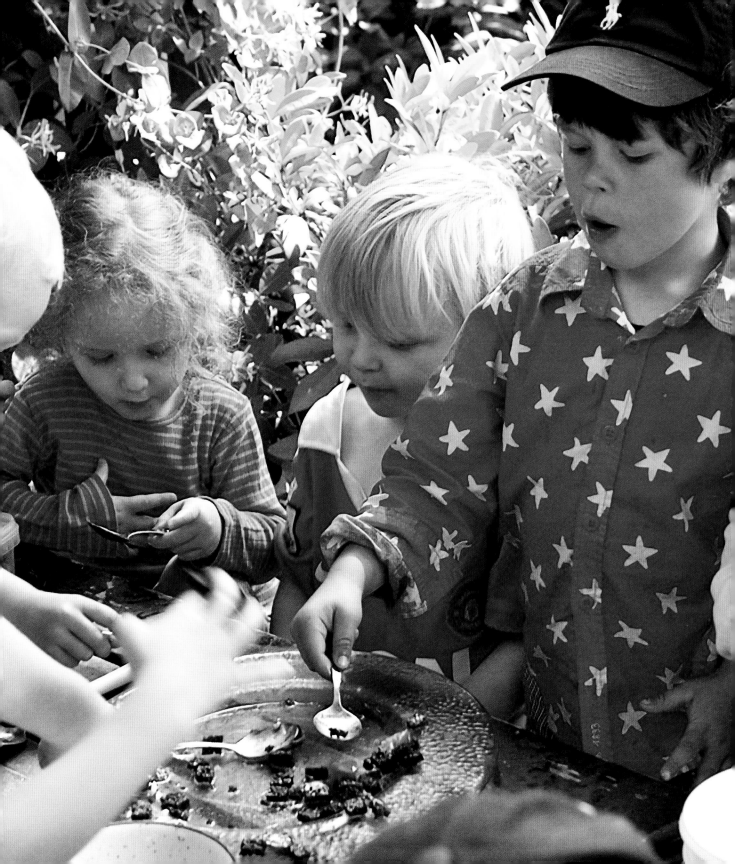

Strawberry vinaigrette with pumpernickel

Our children love these 'rye bread sweets', as we took to calling them. They can, of course, be made separately and enjoyed in all kinds of ways.

Serves a family of 4
3 tbsp maple syrup
10–12 fresh mint leaves
100 ml (½ cup) mint tea or water
½ vanilla pod
6 slices of pumpernickel or other leftover bread
1 punnet of strawberries
2 tbsp neutral oil

Serves 40 children
100 ml (½ cup) maple syrup
1 bunch of fresh mint leaves
250 ml (1 cup) mint tea or water
1 vanilla pod
I kg (2 lb 3 oz) pumpernickel or other leftover bread
8 punnets of local strawberries (approx. 4 kg/8lb 13 oz)
100 ml (½ cup) neutral oil

1. Mix the maple syrup, mint leaves, tea (or water) and the seeds from the vanilla pod in a pan, and heat to make a flavoured syrup. Leave to cool.
2. Cut the bread into small croutons, brush them with oil and syrup.
3. Bake them in the oven for 10 minutes at 180°C (350°F).
4. Hull and slice the strawberries and arrange them on a serving plate. Brush the strawberries with the rest of the syrup and leave to marinate for 15 minutes. Or, if you are making this for a large group, simply toss halved strawberries with syrup.
5. Garnish the strawberries with croutons and serve with whipped cream or crème fraiche.

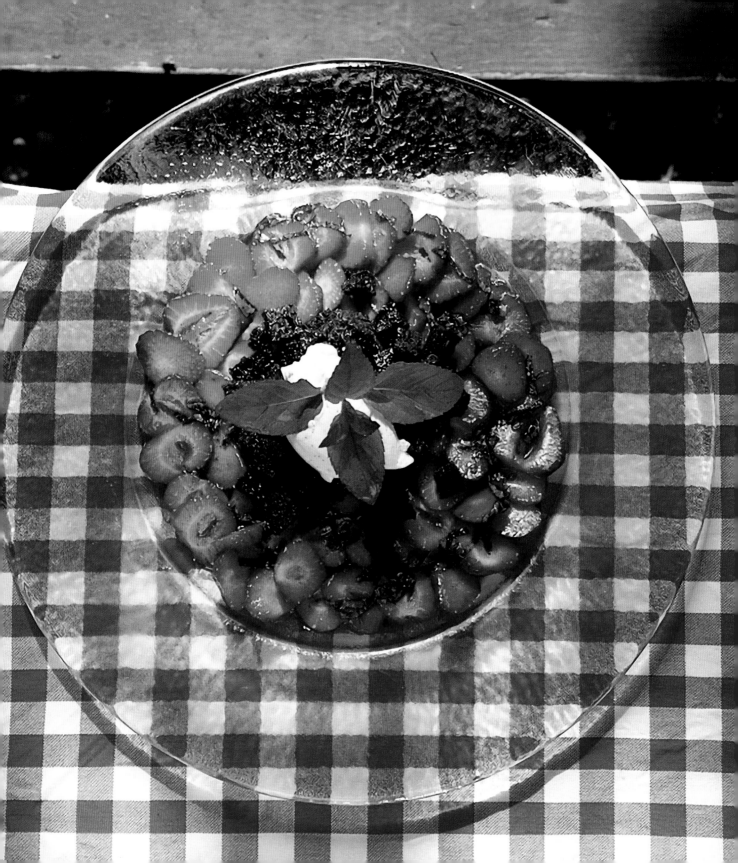

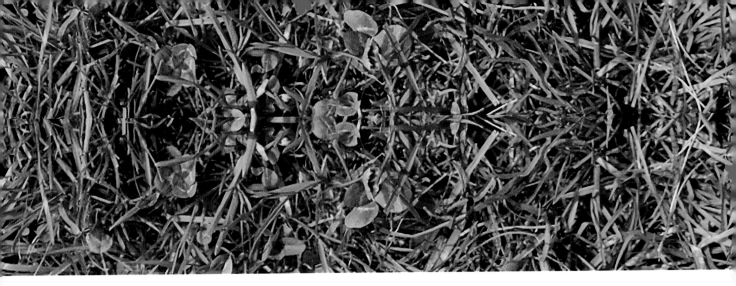

Cherry focaccia

Serves a family of 4
450 g (1 lb) stoned cherries
1 tsp dry yeast
500 ml (1 US pint) lukewarm water
approx. 250 g (9 oz) plain flour
1 tbsp olive oil
50 g (1 ¾ oz) demerara sugar
salt flakes to sprinkle on the bread

Serves 40 children
4 kg (8lb 13 oz) stoned cherries
4 tbsp dry yeast
4 l (8 ½ US pints) lukewarm water
approx. 4.5 kg (9 lb 15 oz) plain flour
4 tbsp olive oil
400 g (14 oz) demerara sugar
salt flakes to sprinkle on the bread

1. Mix the flour, water and yeast to a dough, knead and allow to prove for around 1 hour.
2. Push the dough into a suitable tin, distribute the stoned cherries evenly across the top and let the bread prove for another 30 minutes.
3. Sprinkle the sugar, salt and olive oil onto the bread and bake it at 180°C (350°F) for around 30 minutes, depending on size.

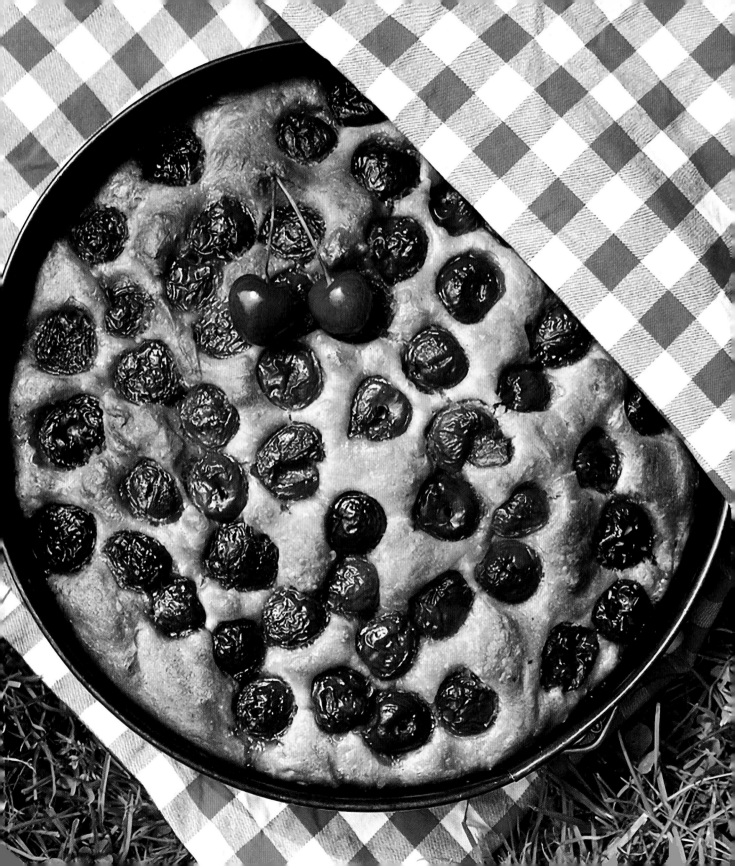

Green pea cake

We were often served this delicious cake on Sundays in L'Osteria di Rendola (Italy), where I lived and worked for a while. My youngest daughter loves the flavour and the crazy green colour. Using frozen peas works well.

Serves 6–8	Serves 40 children
100 g (3 ½ oz) unsalted butter	350 g (12 ⅓ oz) unsalted butter
250 g (9 oz) new onions, chopped	900 g (2 lb) new onions, chopped
2 kg (4 lb 7 oz) peas, hulled (or frozen)	8 kg (17 lb 10 oz) peas, hulled (or frozen)
20 mint leaves, chopped finely	1 large bunch of mint leaves, chopped finely
1 bunch of basil, chopped finely	3 bunches of basil, chopped finely
300 g (10 ½ oz) ricotta cheese	1 kg (2 lb 3 oz) ricotta cheese
4 tbsp whipping cream	250 ml (1 cup) whipping cream
4 large organic eggs	15 large organic eggs
1 tsp herb salt or sea salt	4 tsp herb salt or sea salt
freshly ground black pepper	freshly ground black pepper
juice and zest of 1 organic lemon (optional/to taste)	juice and zest of organic lemons (optional/to taste)
200 g (7 oz) fresh Parmesan cheese	800 g (1 lb 12 oz) fresh Parmesan cheese
olive oil	olive oil

Note: it's not a good idea to use lemon on a daily basis when cooking for a kindergarten because citrus contains a number of allergens. You can leave it out here if you prefer.

1. Sauté the chopped summer onions in the butter.
2. Add the peas and half of the herbs. Leave to simmer for 5 minutes.
3. Pour half of the pea mix into a blender and add the ricotta.
4. Gradually add the cream and eggs.
5. Add the rest of the pea mix and herbs, as well as the lemon juice and zest, and salt and pepper to taste.
6. Grease a cake tin with olive oil and pour in the grated Parmesan. Spread the pea mix on top and bake for 40–45 minutes at 180°C (350°F).

Green pea minestrone

This delicious summer soup is mild and flavoursome. The children can see the ingredients here, which makes a change from always eating blended soups.

Serves a family of 4
150 g (5 ¼ oz) peas, hulled or frozen
2 summer onions
500 g (1 lb 2 oz) new potatoes
2 tbsp olive oil
2 sprigs of thyme
1 l (2 US pints) water
1 tsp herb salt
freshly ground pepper
70 g (2 ½ oz) wholegrain macaroni

Serves 40 children
2 kg (4 lb 7 oz) peas, hulled or frozen
10 summer onions
5 kg (11 lb) new potatoes
200 ml (1 cup) olive oil
1 bunch of thyme
5 l (10 ½ US pints) water
3–4 tsp herb salt
freshly ground pepper
1.5 kg (3 lb 5 oz) wholegrain macaroni

1. Prepare and chop the onions. Scrub and dice the potatoes.
2. Sweat the onions and potatoes in oil in a heavy pan.
3. Add the thyme and water, and let the soup simmer for 15 minutes.
4. Meanwhile, cook the macaroni in lightly salted water for 5–7 minutes (or according to the instructions on the packet).
5. Add the pasta and peas to the soup and season with salt and pepper.
6. Serve straight away with a slice of wholegrain bread.

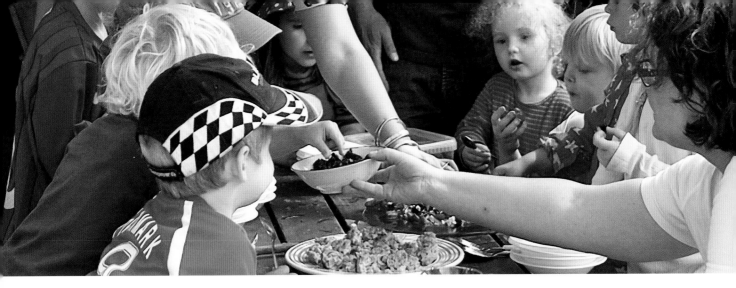

Green pea sandwich spread

As our kindergarten is vegetarian, it's especially important to include enough polyunsaturated fat, selenium and iron in our meal plan, which is why we invented this spread.

Serves 10–15 children
150 g (5 ¼ oz) mung beans
100 ml (½ cup) thistle oil
65 g (2 ⅓ oz) sunflower seeds
150g (5 ¼ oz) green peas, fresh or frozen
100 ml (½ cup) boiling water
1 tsp herb salt
1 tbsp white balsamic vinegar

1. Boil the mung beans until soft (around 25 minutes, no pre-soaking required).
2. Mix the beans the with oil, sunflower seeds and peas and blend to a smooth paste.
3. Add boiling water until the paste spreads easily.
4. Season the spread with salt and vinegar, and serve on rye bread or wholegrain bread.

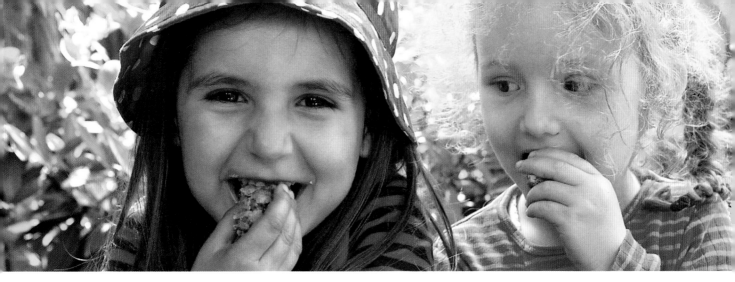

Dill cucumbers

When cucumbers are delivered to Bonsai, it's always set to be an exciting day. The children play for hours with 'green snakes' and 'wild monsters'. The teachers might tell a story about the adventures of the cucumbers, and then we eat them with a dill dressing.

Serves a family of 4
1 cucumber
2 tsp herb salt
7 tbsp buttermilk
1 tsp Dijon mustard
3 sprigs of dill

Serves 40 children
10 cucumbers
5 tsp herb salt
750 ml (1½ US pints) buttermilk
4 tsp Dijon mustard
1 bunch of dill

1. Halve the cucumber lengthwise and slice it thinly. Sprinkle with salt and leave for roughly an hour to draw out some of the water.
2. Meanwhile, mix the buttermilk, mustard and finely chopped dill.
3. Rinse the cucumber slices and dry them with a cloth.
4. Toss the cucumber with the dressing and serve as a side dish or dip.

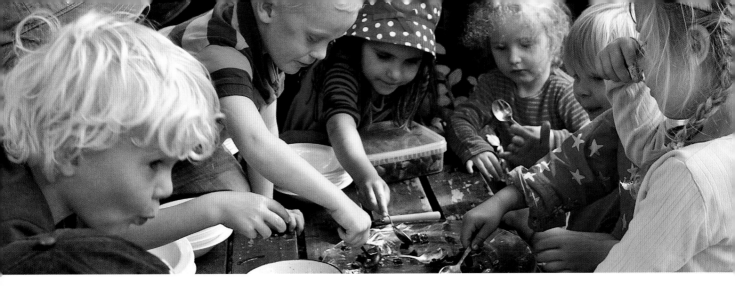

Pickled cucumbers

Our suppliers often provide produce, such as cucumbers, in large quantities, so we pickle them to avoid waste. The children love cutting the cucumbers into shapes using cookie cutters. It's fun to be served your own home-pickled cucumber star!

Makes pickling liquid for 7–8 cucumbers
500 ml (1 US pint) vinegar
500 g (1lb 2 oz) demerara sugar
1 l (2 US pints) water

Bouquet garni (you can use a self-fill tea bag)
2 star anise pods
1 tsp pink peppercorns
1 tsp coriander seeds
1 tsp herb salt

1. Bring the water, vinegar and sugar to the boil.
2. Slice the cucumbers and put them in a big sterilised picking jar.
3. Pour over the liquid and add the bouquet garni.
4. Leave to infuse for some time before eating.

If you take the jar straight from the dishwasher and boil it in water for a few minutes after sealing it, there's no need to use preservatives.

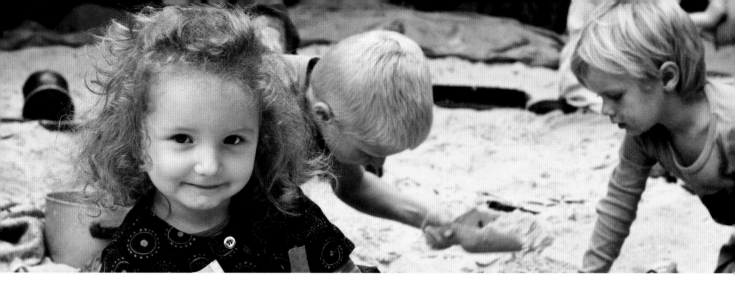

Cucumber and melon soup

This delicate summer soup is delicious served hot or cold.

Serves a family of 4
2 onions
2 celery stalks
3 carrots
2 tbsp oil
1 clove of garlic
3 tbsp basmati rice
3 tbsp organic coconut milk
1 large glass of herbal tea
1 cucumber
½ Galia melon

Serves 40 children
12 summer onions
2 bunches of celery stalks
2.5 kg (5 lb 8 oz) carrots
300 ml (1 ¼ cups) oil
8 cloves of garlic
1.5 kg (3 lb 5 oz) basmati rice
2 cans of organic coconut milk
1 l (2 US pints) herbal tea
6 cucumbers
3 Galia melons

1. Prepare the fruit and vegetables and cut them into thick slices.
2. Boil all the ingredients, except the cucumber and melon, until soft (around 30 minutes).
3. Leave the soup to cool a little before mixing in the cucumber and melon.
4. You may want to refrigerate the soup for a few hours, unless you're planning to serve it hot. Serve with bread.

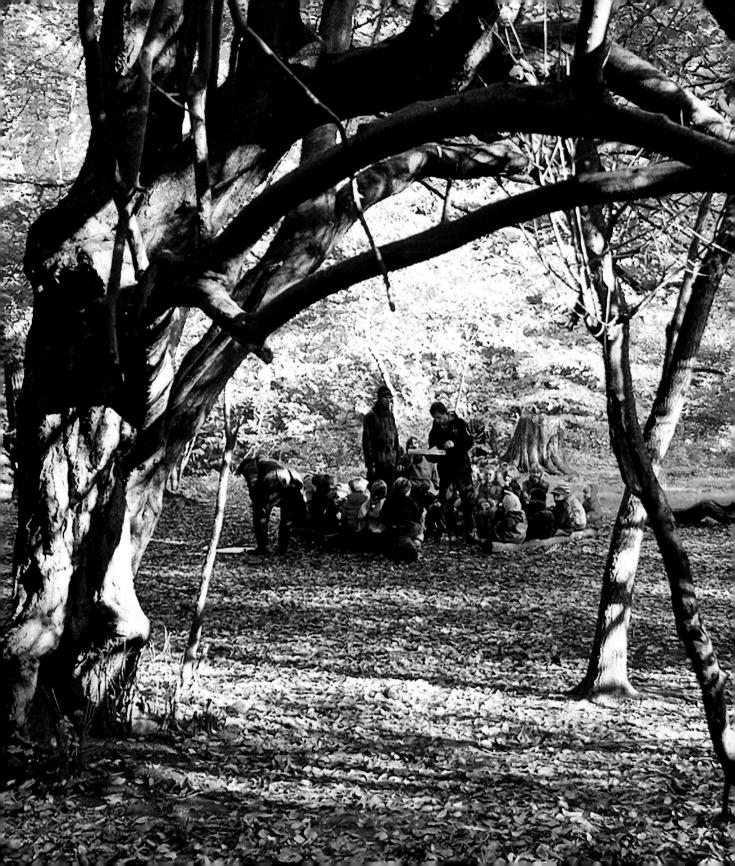

Autumn

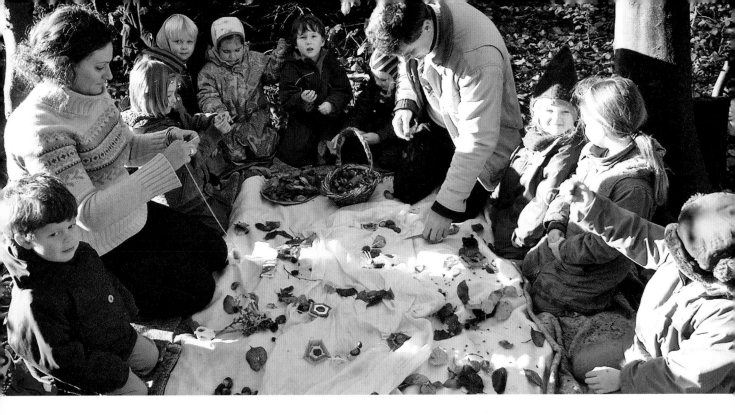

While spring and summer are characterised by extroversion, outdoor activities and sweet vegetables, autumn calls for inward reflection, fires and soup.

Nature is particularly powerful in the autumn. Go for a walk in the woods and you will see a magical explosion of colour in reds, yellows and browns. Autumn brings wind, rain and storms as well as sun and blue skies. It is breathtaking and invigorating.

Although we associate autumn with decay, this is a necessary evil in the seasonal cycle, which provides a welcome contrast to delicate spring and exuberant summer. When considered together, the year with its different seasons is an organic whole. It's worth remembering when we're stuck with autumn-wet socks and winter-cold cheeks that we can enjoy everything nature has to offer.

That's why we pride ourselves on using seasonal ingredients and living in harmony with nature. In fact, it's a great way of practising mindfulness – in relation to ourselves and our environment. In northern Europe, autumn brings juicy root vegetables, full of flavour and nutrients, and rustic cereals with their unique qualities. These become our focus now, and thanks to them there is no reason to yearn for the sun-ripened tomatoes and crisp lettuce of summer, because autumn gives us everything we need.

At Bonsai this means we gradually turn to warm, rich soups, which will become even more common during winter. We start to use big pans on the hob, or even better, over an open fire: our favourite method of cooking whenever the weather allows it. We pick gorgeous mushrooms in the forest, brimming with protein. We roast

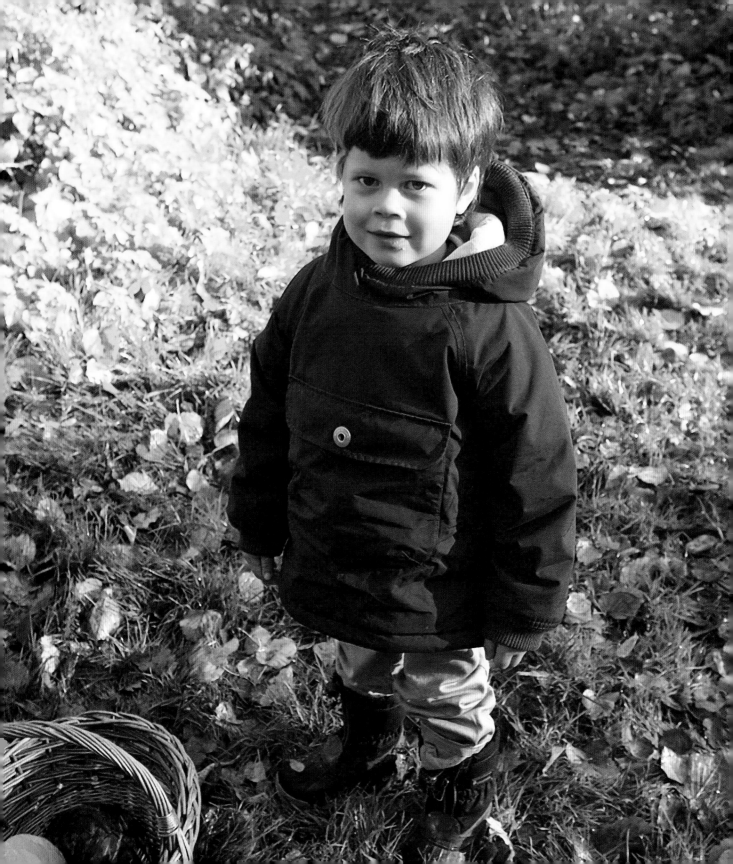

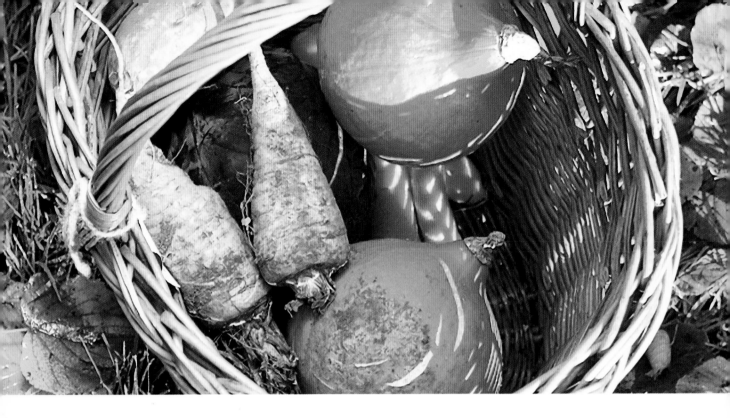

or pickle them or turn them into pâté, which we eat with the lovely, homemade bread that accompanies every meal from now until the other side of winter.

Like the animals of the forest, we gather acorns, conkers, elderberries, apples, blackberries, rosehips, rowan berries, leaves and branches.

We use what we find creatively to bring nature indoors, in the shape of animals made from conkers, berry and rosehip garlands, acorn fairies, beautiful nuts in a decorative bowl and gorgeous wreaths made of fallen leaves. All these activities encourage contemplation, serenity and mindfulness.

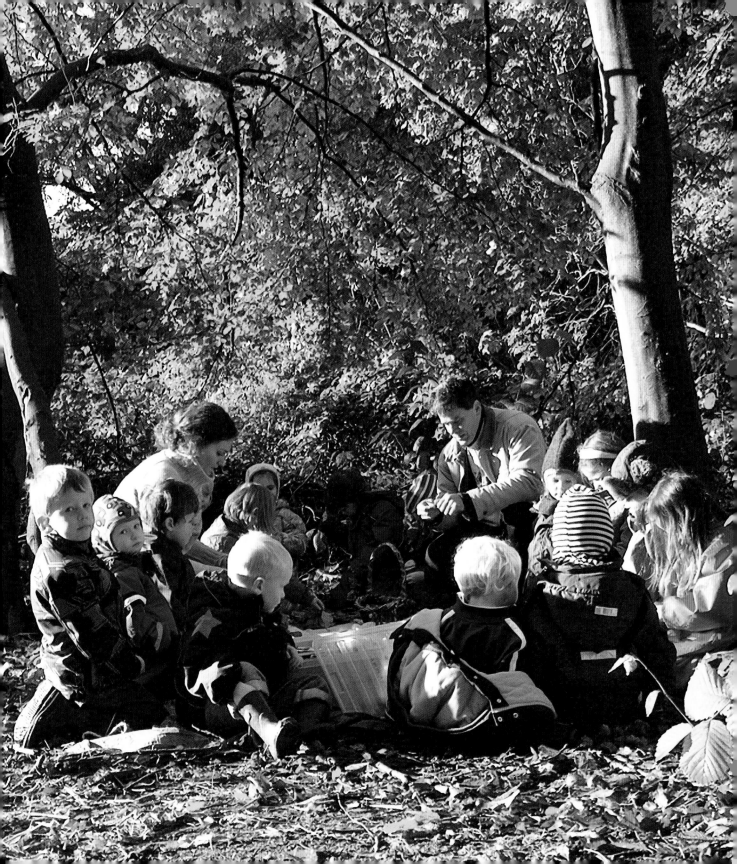

Chilli con tofu

Many children love mince, but this vegetarian chilli will also hit the mark, once the little ones have got used to it.

Serves a family of 4
2 onions, grated or finely chopped
1 clove of garlic, finely chopped
200 g (7 oz) green beans
a splash of oil
150 g (5¼ oz) cooked kidney beans
1 tsp paprika
a pinch of chilli or cayenne pepper
1 packet of marinated tofu
1 tsp Dijon mustard
a splash of maple syrup
sea salt or herb salt

Serves 40 children
7–8 onions, grated or finely chopped
3–4 cloves of garlic, finely chopped
1 kg (2 lb 3 oz) green beans
100 ml (½ cup) oil
2.5 kg (5 lb 8 oz) cooked kidney beans
2 tsp paprika
a pinch of chilli or cayenne pepper
6 packets of marinated tofu
a dollop of Dijon mustard
2 tbsp maple syrup
sea salt or herb salt

1. Trim the green beans and blanch them in lightly salted water for a few minutes; they should still be crunchy. Cut them into bite-sized pieces.
2. Chop or grate the onions and garlic and sweat them in oil in a heavy pan.
3. Add the kidney beans and seasoning and leave to simmer for 10 minutes.
4. Dice the tofu and add to the pan.
5. Add the mustard, maple syrup and salt to taste, then stir in the blanched green beans.
6. Serve with rice, bread and crème fraiche.

Note: dried beans need to be pre-soaked in water overnight and precooked in fresh water. If you're short on time, you can use organic, precooked tinned beans.

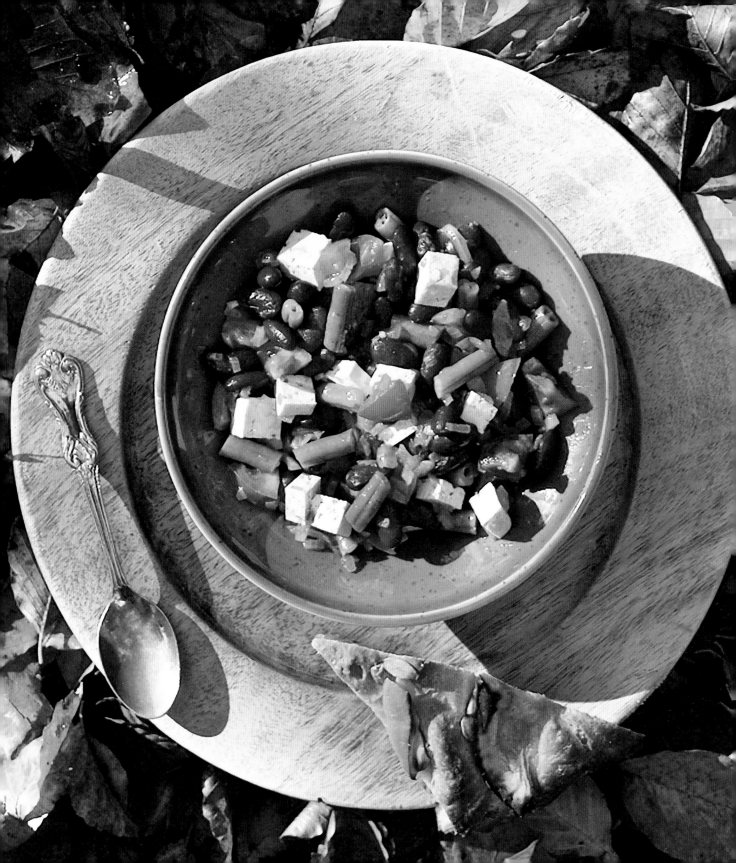

Pom's Asian bean salad

At the fish restaurant, Skagen, I worked with a Thai monk called Pom. Rarely have I seen such mindfulness during vegetable prep. He used a toothbrush to clean lettuce and leafy greens, and I have never again, in all my working life, seen vegetables prepared with such love and care.

Serves a family of 4
250 g (9 oz) green beans
1 red pepper
3 tbsp toasted coconut flakes
2 tbsp roasted peanuts

Dressing
juice and zest of ½ organic lemon
2 tbsp peanut or sesame oil
pinch of sea salt

Serves 40 children
2.5 kg (5 lb 8 oz) green beans
3–4 red peppers
9 tbsp toasted coconut flakes
10 tbsp roasted peanuts

Dressing
juice and zest of 2 organic lemons
200 ml (1 cup) peanut or sesame oil
pinch of sea salt

1. Trim the beans and boil them until al dente in lightly salted water. Rinse them in cold water to help retain their bright green colour.
2. Deseed the peppers and dice them finely.
3. Mix the ingredients for the dressing and season to taste.
4. Toast the coconut lightly in a dry pan, then do the same with the peanuts.
5. Toss the peppers and beans with the dressing and top with the coconut and peanuts.

You can make your own coconut flakes from a fresh coconut using a julienne peeler. The salad tastes best with peanuts you have cracked yourself and roasted in a hot pan. Both the cracking and the frying are great tasks for children. But if they're busy playing football and you're in a hurry, you can use ready-to-eat peanuts and coconut from the shop.

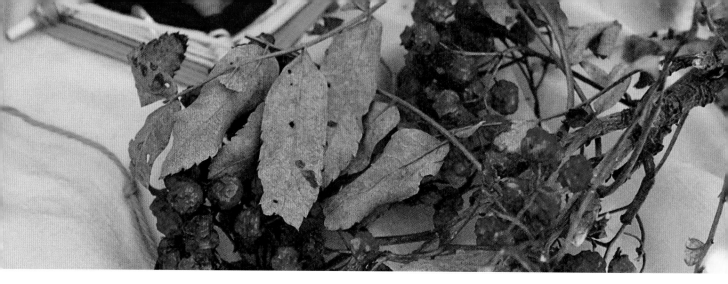

Squash and white bean sandwich spread

Serves a family of 4

1 kg (2 lb 3 oz) white beans (of any kind)
1 large red kuri (or butternut) squash, peeled and deseeded
100 ml (½ cup) olive oil
200–300 ml (1–1 ¼ cups) boiling water (not the water from the beans!)
sea salt
freshly ground pepper
2 tbsp crushed fennel seeds
zest and juice of 1 organic orange

1. Soak the white beans overnight. Drain and cook in fresh water for around 45 minutes or until completely soft.
2. Dice the squash roughly and roast at 200°C (400°F) for 25 minutes.
3. Mix the beans and squash with the olive oil and boiling water.
4. Add salt and pepper to taste and mix in the fennel seeds, orange juice and zest.
5. Pour the spread into a pretty tin lined with cling film and refrigerate until set.

You can also use the spread as a soup base, and it freezes well.

Pickled squash

Squash is a beautiful vegetable that can be used in many ways: first to decorate your table or windowsill; then in a delicious soup. And pickled squash makes a great alternative to cucumber in lunch boxes. It makes sense to make a big batch, even if there are only four or five of you in the house.

Serves a family of 4

½ red kuri squash (or another variety of squash, such as butternut)

Pickling liquid
250 ml (1 cup) organic pickling vinegar
100 ml (½ cup) water
75 g (2 ⅔ oz) demerara sugar
1 star anise pod
juice and zest of ½ organic lemon

Serves 40 children

5–6 red kuri squashes (or another variety of squash, such as butternut)

Pickling liquid
2 l (4 ¼ US pints) organic pickling vinegar
1 l (2 US pints) water
750 g (1 lb 10 oz) demerara sugar
5 star anise pods
juice and zest of 2 organic lemons

1. Peel the squash, remove the seeds and dice it.
2. Put all the ingredients for the pickling liquid in a pot and bring to the boil.
3. Add the diced squash to the boiling liquid and take it off the heat. Leave everything to cool completely.
4. Then pour the squash and liquid into clean, sterilised pickling jars.

You can, of course, use preservatives to ensure the longevity of the pickled squash. But if you prefer not to use preservatives, you can wash the pickling jars in the dishwasher instead and only take them out when you are ready to use them. Then pour the squash in, seal the lid and finish by boiling the sealed jars in water for a few minutes.

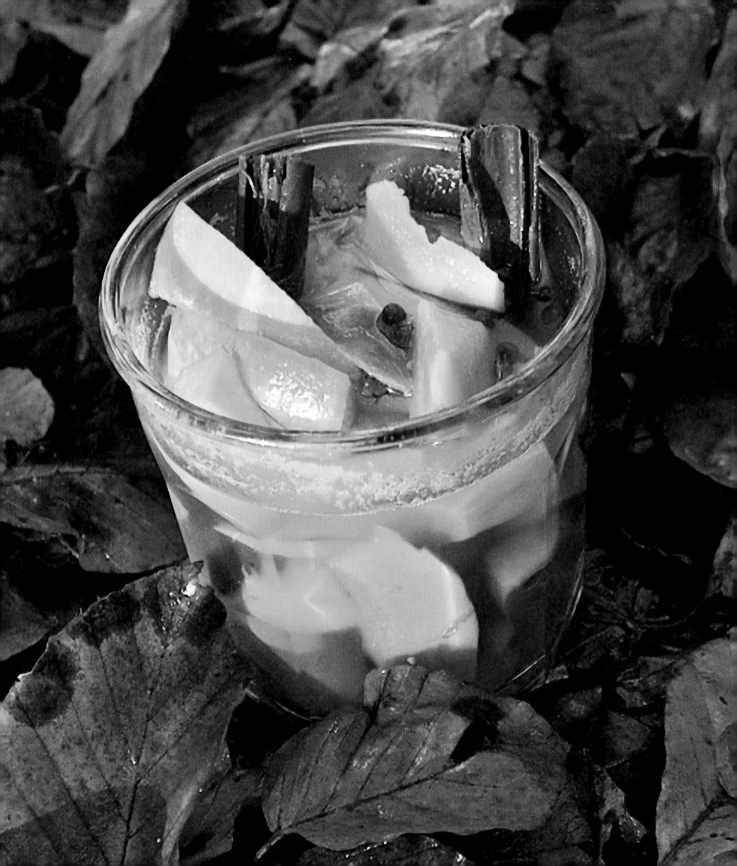

Autumn bread with squash

Serves a family of 4
7 g (¼ oz) fresh yeast
750 ml (1½ US pints) lukewarm water
750–800 g (1 lb 10–12 oz) Öland wheat flour
45 g (1½ oz) bran
1 tsp salt
1 tsp honey
¼ red kuri (or butternut) squash, peeled,
  deseeded and diced
2 tbsp squash seeds

Serves 40 children
25 g (1 oz) fresh yeast
3 l (6 ⅓ US pints) lukewarm water
3 kg (6 lb 10 oz) Öland wheat flour
275 g (9 ½ oz) bran
1 tbsp salt
1 tbsp honey
2 red kuri (or butternut) squashes, peeled,
  deseeded and diced
2 handfuls of squash seeds

1. Dissolve the yeast in the water and add the flour and bran.
2. Knead well. Then add salt and honey and knead again.
3. Leave the dough to prove overnight in the fridge.
4. Tip the dough onto a baking tray lined with greaseproof paper. Press the squash pieces gently into the dough so they stick up slightly, decorating the bread. Sprinkle the seeds over the bread.
5. Bake at 200°C (400°F) for 30 minutes.

If the bread is for children under the age of three, you should dice the squash finely.

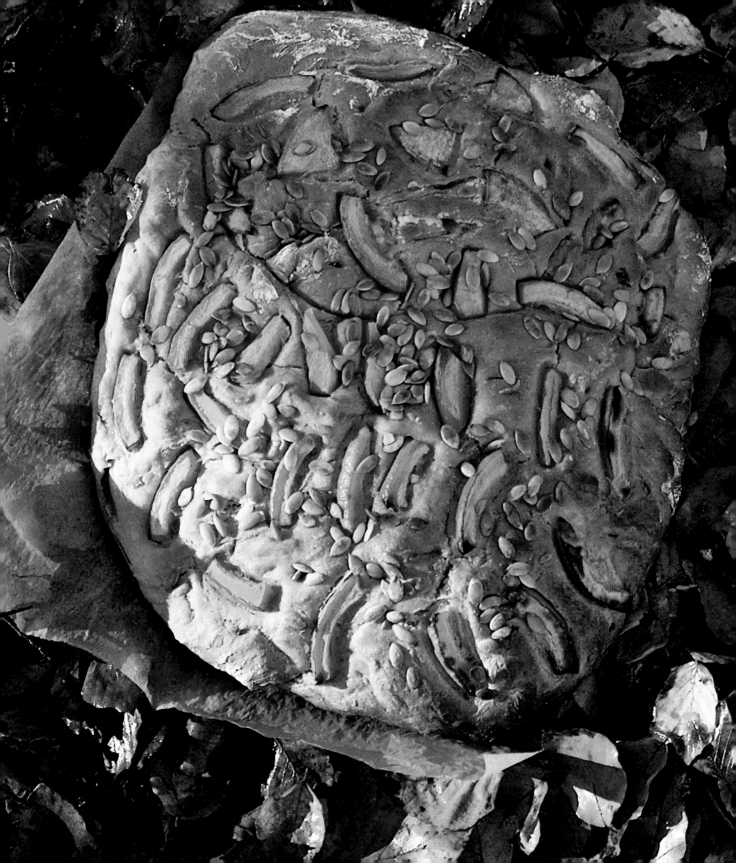

Mild pumpkin curry.

This mild but very nutritious curry makes the perfect outdoor stew on a dreary autumn day.

Serves a family of 4

1 red kuri or butternut squash, or other variety
  of small pumpkin
1 sweet potato or carrot
1 tsp madras curry powder
1 tsp fresh ginger, chopped
1 clove of garlic
1 onion, finely chopped
splash of oil
500 ml (1 US pint) water
½ can of organic coconut milk (optional)
200g (7oz) precooked chickpeas
sea salt
freshly ground pepper

Serves 40 children

5–6 red kuri or butternut squashes, or other
  variety of small pumpkin
2 kg (4 lb 7 oz) sweet potato or carrot
2 tbsp madras curry powder
1 tbsp fresh ginger, chopped
5 cloves of garlic
8 onions, finely chopped
100 ml (½ cup) oil
7 l (14 ¾ US pints) water
1 can of organic coconut milk (optional)
2.5 kg (5 ½ lb) precooked chickpeas
sea salt
freshly ground pepper

1. Prepare the squash and sweet potato or carrot and cut them into bite-sized pieces, roughly the same size.
2. Sweat the curry powder, ginger, garlic and onion in oil in a heavy pan.
3. Add the vegetables and let them fry for a moment before adding the water and coconut milk (if using). Leave to simmer for 20 minutes.
4. Stir in the chickpeas and cook for another 10 minutes.
5. Finally add salt and pepper to taste.
6. You could garnish the curry with finely chopped blanched kale and serve with brown rice or wholegrain bread.

Pumpkin soup

Serves a family of 4

1 red kuri or butternut squash, or other variety
  of small pumpkin
1 onion
3–4 large potatoes
3 carrots
2 tsp oil
1 clove of garlic
pinch of chopped fresh ginger
½ tsp cayenne pepper
1 tsp herb salt or sea salt
1.5 l (3 US pints) water
1 can of organic coconut milk

Serves 40 children

7 red kuri or butternut squashes, or other
  variety of small pumpkin
7 onions
20 large potatoes
15 carrots
100 ml (½ cup) oil
5 cloves of garlic
2 tsp chopped fresh ginger
2 tsp cayenne pepper
2 tsp herb salt or sea salt
8 l (17 US pints) water
3 cans of organic coconut milk

1. Prepare all the vegetables and dice them roughly. Sweat them in oil in a heavy pot.
2. Add the garlic, ginger, salt and cayenne pepper.
3. Pour in the water and allow to simmer for half an hour.
4. Blend the soup well and stir in the coconut milk. Leave the soup to simmer for another 10–15 minutes.
5. Add salt to taste, and serve with autumn (see p. 100) or wholegrain bread.

Let the children help you with the squash; they love digging out the seeds. If you have time, you can sprinkle the seeds with salt and dry them in the oven.

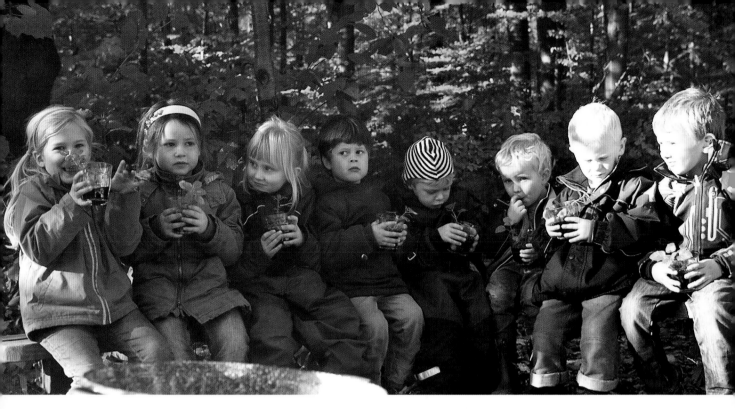

Herb tea

You can make delicious tea over the campfire using fresh or dried herbs, such as mint, sage and liquorice root. Or how about some elderflower squash (see p. 62) or a rich, warm cup of hot chocolate?

At Bonsai we have a small herb garden, which means we can pick herbs straight from the garden to put in our tea. Picking the herbs yourself makes the tea even tastier, especially for the children!

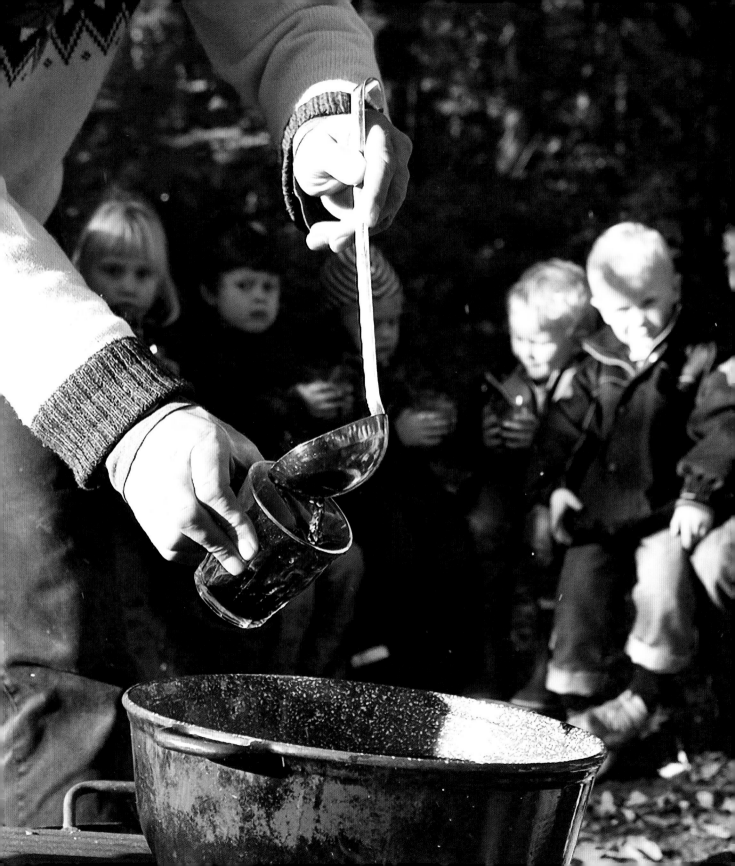

Carsten's *svedjerug* bread

Svedjerug is an ancient variety of rye, discovered in the seventies in Norway. The grain is particularly good for baking and has a wonderfully aromatic flavour. Svedjerug is challenging to cultivate because the grains are small and the stalks are long, which makes it particularly vulnerable to heavy rain. Yields of svedjerug are significantly less plentiful than those of modern rye.

During the summer of 2010, my children and I were given the opportunity to help harvest svedjerug at a local biodynamic farm. The farmers, Carsten and Rikke Hvelplund Jensen, even let us drive the combine harvester, which was a very special experience.

Makes 2 loaves

Day 1
750 ml (1 ½ US pints) lukewarm water
50 g (1 ¾ oz) sourdough starter (available from
 health-food shops)

75 g (2 ⅓ oz) cracked rye
1 tbsp salt
1 tsp honey
450 g (1 lb) *svedjerug* flour

1. Mix all the ingredients in a bowl, cover with a cloth and leave to rest overnight.

Day 2
1 l (2 US pints) water
775 g (1 lb 11 oz) *svedjerug* flour
450 g (1 lb) spelt flour

1. Stir the new ingredients into the dough.
2. Knead it well and divide between 2 greased bread tins, approx. 900 g (2 lb) per tin.
3. Prick the loaves with a fork and brush with water, then leave to prove for at least 2 hours.
4. Bake at 200°C (400°F) for around 1¼ hours.
5. Then lower the temperature to 180°C (350°F), remove the bread tins and leave the loaves to bake for another 30 minutes or so. Their core temperature should be 98°C (200°F). You can measure the temperature by inserting an oven thermometer into the middle of the loaf.
6. Let the loaves cool on a rack, then store in a cool place, wrapped in cloth inside plastic bags.

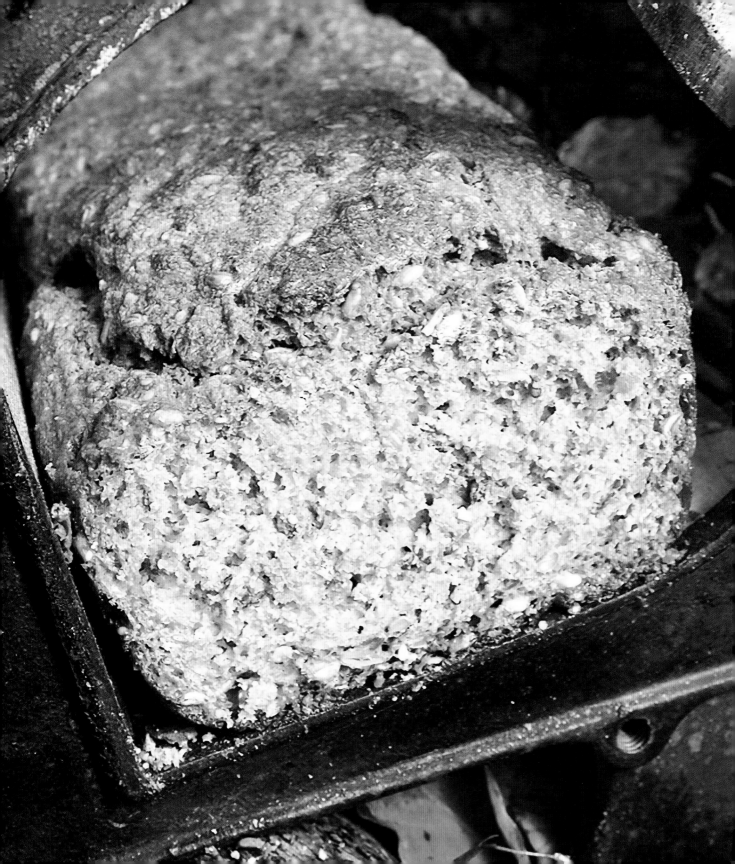

Cured cabbage

This raw dish is great because the salt makes the cabbage both crispy and tender, so even small children can eat it. This cured cabbage can be added to practically any type of side dish; whatever you can find in your cupboards.

Serves a family of 4
½ white cabbage
2 tbsp herb salt or sea salt

Serves 40 children
5 large white cabbages (or 3 white cabbages and
  2 savoy cabbages)
8 tbsp herb salt or sea salt

1. Slice the cabbage thinly, preferably on a mandolin.
2. Mix with the salt and leave for at least 2 hours before rinsing thoroughly and drying on a cloth.

With pickled squash
Slice the pickled squash thinly, add the cured cabbage and toss with a vinaigrette.

With pears and hazelnuts
1. Toast chopped hazelnuts in 2 tbsp oil in a hot frying pan, then add 1 tbsp white balsamic vinegar and bring to the boil. Shake to coat the nuts.
2. Toss with cured cabbage, sliced pears and fennel seeds.

With apples and dried cranberries
1. Make a vinaigrette and drizzle over the cranberries.
2. Core some apples and cut them into rings.
3. Toss the cabbage, apples, cranberries and dressing.

Dressing suggestions
• Shake 300 ml (1¼ cups) quality oil with 100 ml (½ cup) vinegar, and add sea salt and pepper to taste.
• Mix 400 ml (1⅔ cups) buttermilk with 1 tbsp mustard, and add sea salt and pepper to taste.

Grandma's cabbage rolls

Cabbage rolls are a wonderful, old-fashioned dish. Most children love making them – and eating them, of course!

Serves a family of 4

8 large savoy cabbage leaves
250 g (9 oz) boiled chickpeas (can be tinned)
1 onion, finely chopped
1 clove of garlic, finely chopped
1 carrot, grated
splash of oil
1 tsp sea salt or herb salt
juice and zest of ¼ organic lemon
1 tsp garam masala
freshly ground black pepper

Serves 40 children

50 large savoy cabbage leaves
1.5 kg (3 lb 5 oz) boiled chickpeas
  (can be tinned)
7 onions, finely chopped
5 cloves of garlic, finely chopped
9 carrots, grated
100 ml (½ cup) oil
2 tbsp sea salt or herb salt
juice and zest of 1 organic lemon
4 tbsp garam masala
freshly ground black pepper

1. Blanch the cabbage leaves in boiling water for around 1 minute, depending on size, then take the leaves out and rinse them in cold water.
2. Blend the chickpeas coarsely.
3. Fry the onion, garlic and carrot in oil until golden.
4. Add the chickpeas, salt, pepper, lemon and garam masala.
5. Line up the blanched cabbage leaves and place 1 tbsp of filling on each. Roll each leaf and secure with string or toothpicks.
6. Fry them in oil and season with salt and pepper.

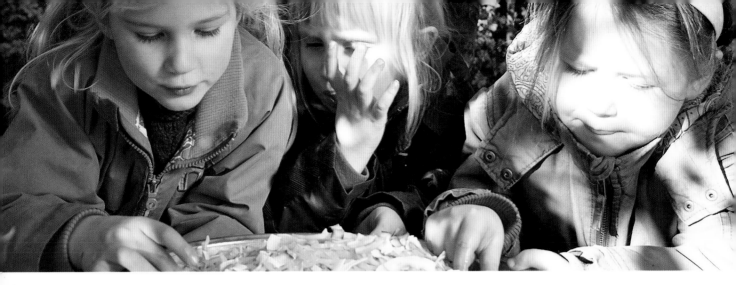

Cabbage curry

This quick cabbage dish tastes great and works well as a main course.

Serves a family of 4
¼ white cabbage
1 apple
splash of oil
1 tsp madras curry powder
½ can of organic coconut milk
pinch of sea salt or herb salt
2 handfuls of flaked coconut

Serves 40 children
5 small white cabbages
5 apples
1 tbsp oil
2–3 tbsp madras curry powder
3 cans of organic coconut milk
2 tsp sea salt or herb salt
200 g (7 oz) flaked coconut

1. Slice the cabbage and apples thinly.
2. Heat the oil in a wok or frying pan. Fry the curry powder quickly then add the apple, cabbage and coconut milk.
3. Leave to boil for 3–4 minutes, then add salt to taste.
4. You can make your own coconut flakes from a fresh coconut using a julienne peeler, or you can buy them ready-made. Roast the coconut flakes in the oven until golden to really bring out the flavour. Sprinkle them over the curry.

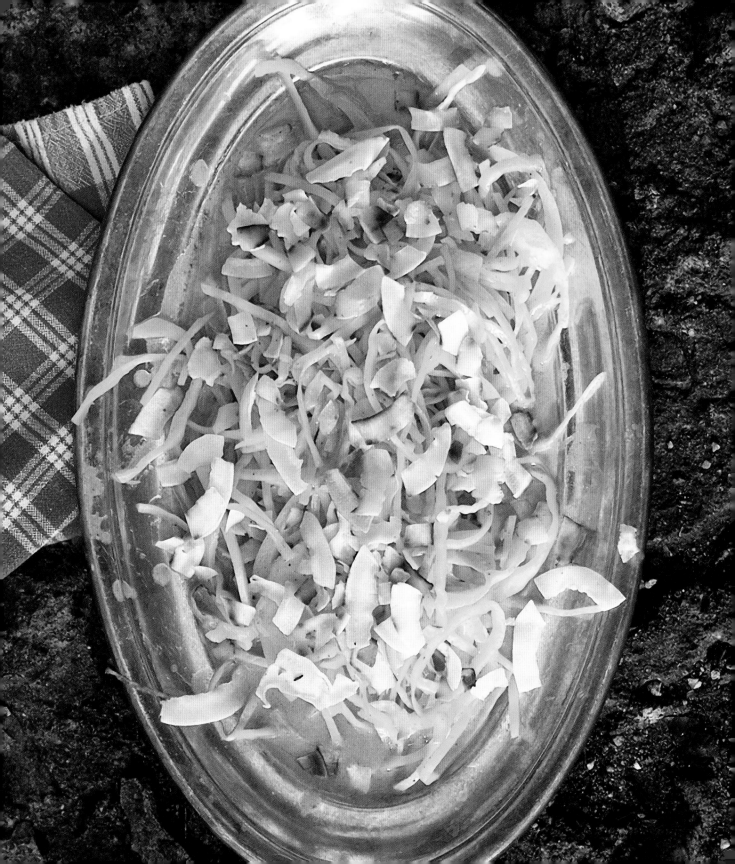

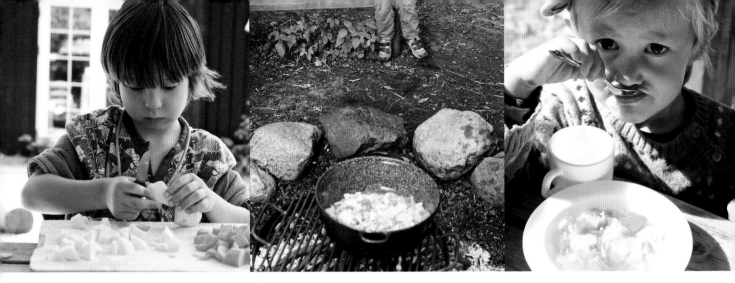

Jesper's campfire soup

Children like nothing more than helping out with cooking, especially around the fire in the garden. So get them working! Peeling and chopping are great jobs for children.

Serves 17 children and 2 adults
2 onions
½ white cabbage
10 large potatoes
1 large sweet potato
8 carrots
100 ml (½ cup) oil
1 cinnamon stick
1.5 l (3 US pints) water
sea salt
freshly ground pepper
handful of fresh, chopped mint leaves

1. Prepare the vegetables and slice them thinly.
2. Hang a pot over the fire and add the oil. Fry the vegetables and add the cinnamon stick.
3. Pour in the water and leave the soup to simmer for half an hour.
4. Add salt and pepper to taste and finish the soup with mint.

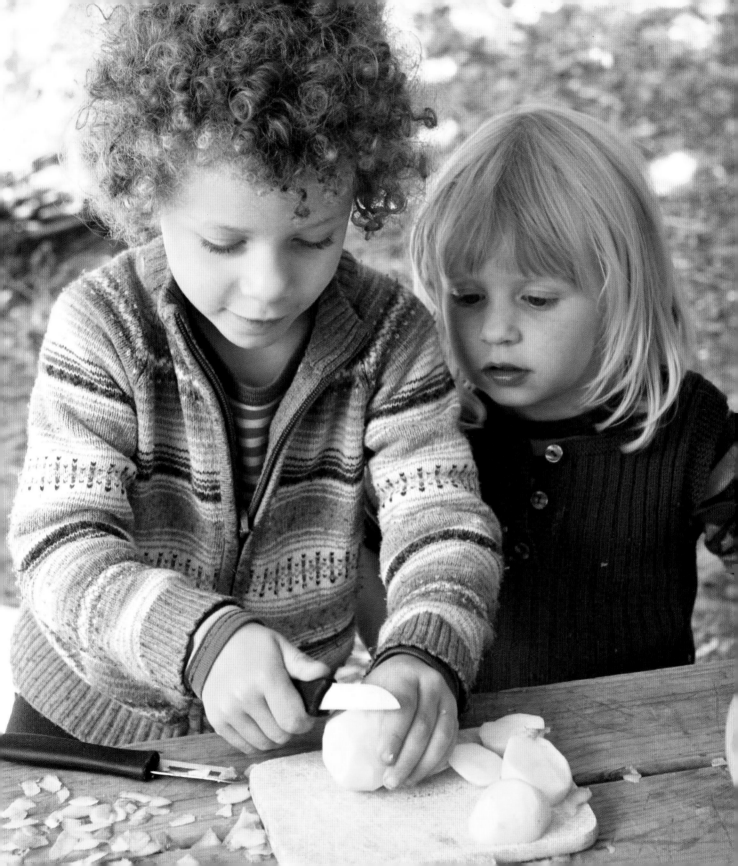

Preserved autumn mushrooms

Going mushroom picking gives you a great reason to go exploring in the woods. However, if you're not 100 per cent sure which mushrooms are edible and which aren't, it's safer to pay a visit to your local greengrocer.

To fill a 2.5 l (5 ¼ US pint) pickling jar
1 kg (2 lb 3 oz) mixed mushrooms
3 tsp herb salt or sea salt
1 tsp fennel seeds
juice and zest of 2 organic lemons
2–3 bay leaves
700 ml (1½ US pints) thistle or sunflower oil

1. Clean the mushrooms thoroughly and cut them into smaller pieces.
2. Put the herb salt, fennel seeds and lemon zest in a mortar and grind.
3. Sprinkle the mix over the mushrooms and put everything in a sterilised pickling jar. Jars taken straight from the dishwasher will be sterile.
4. Heat the oil almost to boiling in a pan and carefully pour it over the mushrooms. Add the bay leaves.
5. Leave the jar to cool uncovered, then seal and refrigerate.
6. The mushrooms can be stored for up to 2 months.

Preserved mushrooms make a great addition to pasta, risotto, soup and various sauces, and can be used to liven up sandwiches.

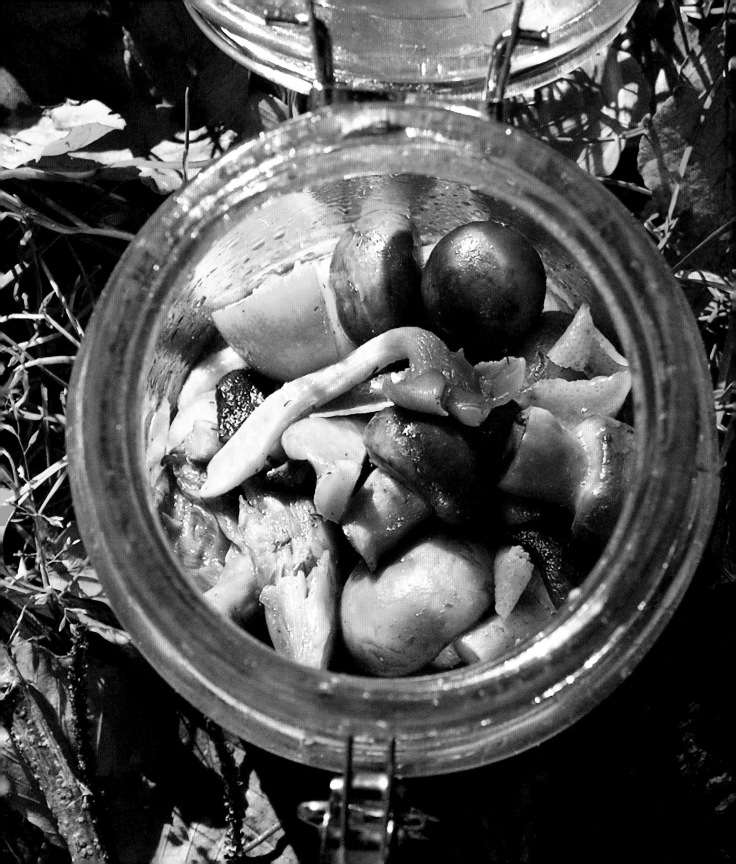

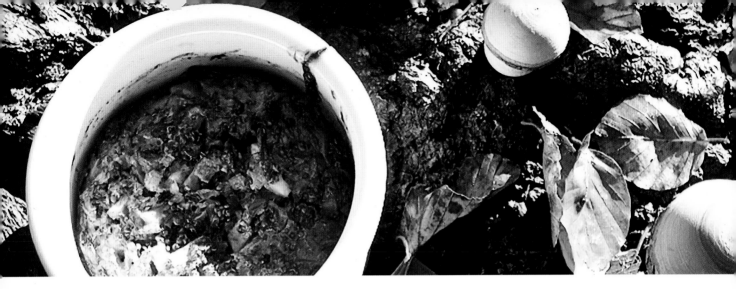

Mushroom pâté

250 g (9 oz) onion, finely chopped
1 tbsp olive oil
500 g (1 lb 2 oz) mixed
  mushrooms, chopped
approx. 170g boiled rice or lentils
  (leftovers work well here)
1 clove of garlic, finely chopped

1 tbsp crushed fennel seeds
1 tbsp finely chopped fresh
  thyme (or dried thyme)
1 tsp herb salt or sea salt
2 organic eggs
75 ml (⅓ cup) buttermilk
150 ml (⅔ cup) water

1. Fry the onions first in oil in a hot pan, then the mushrooms. Set aside to cool.
2. Mix the sautéed vegetables with the rest of the ingredients, and pour the mix into a tin, approx. 15 x 30cm (6 x 12 inches).
3. Bake the pâté at 180°C (350°F) for around 30 minutes. It should feel firm when you prick it.

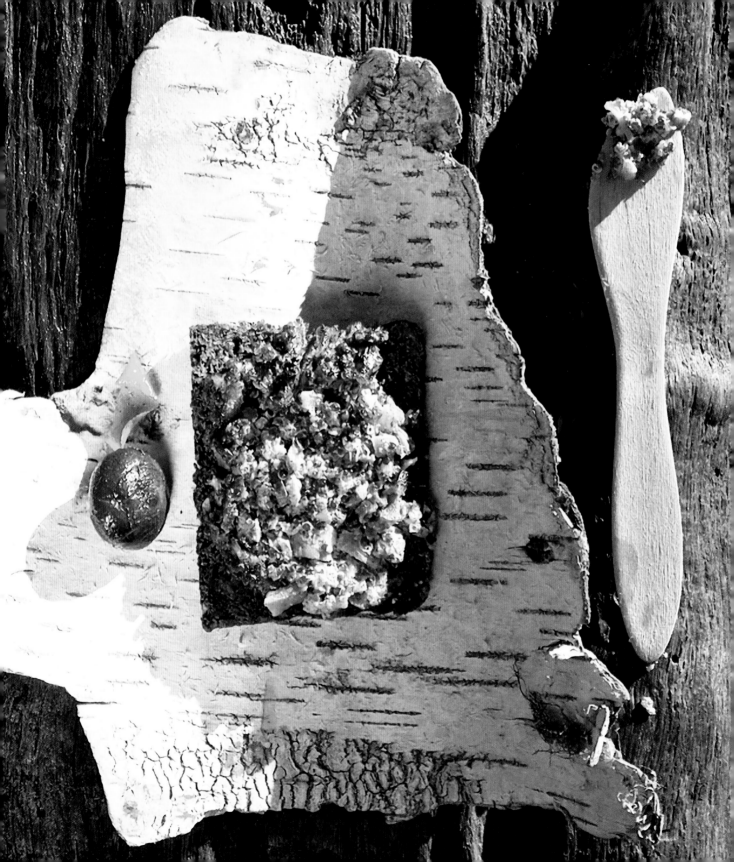

Mushroom soup

Serves a family of 4
250 g (9 oz) mixed mushrooms
½ celeriac
3 large potatoes
1 onion
1 clove of garlic
1 tsp oil
½ tsp thyme
½ tsp Dijon mustard
¼ can of organic coconut milk
water
herb salt or sea salt
freshly ground pepper

Serves 40 children
1 kg (2 lb 3 oz) mixed mushrooms
2 celeriac
5 kg (11 lb) large potatoes
4 onions
2 cloves of garlic
2 tbsp oil
1 tbsp thyme
1 tbsp Dijon mustard
1 can of organic coconut milk
water
herb salt or sea salt
freshly ground pepper

Garnish
rye bread for crispy croutons
a few drops of balsamic vinegar

1. Peel the celeriac and potatoes and chop roughly. Chop the onion and garlic.
2. Clean the mushrooms. Take a quarter of the best-looking mushrooms and set them aside for the garnish.
3. Fry the vegetables in oil in a large pot.
4. Add water to cover the vegetables and leave to cook for 45 minutes.
5. Add the coconut milk, mustard and thyme, and leave to simmer.
6. Finally add the salt and pepper to taste and blend until smooth and creamy.
7. Fry small rye bread croutons in butter or oil until crispy.
8. Chop the rest of the mushrooms, especially if cooking for children, and fry them quickly in a very hot pan.
9. Sprinkle the mushrooms with a few drops of balsamic vinegar and some salt and pepper.
10. Pour the soup into bowls, adding a spoonful of each topping.

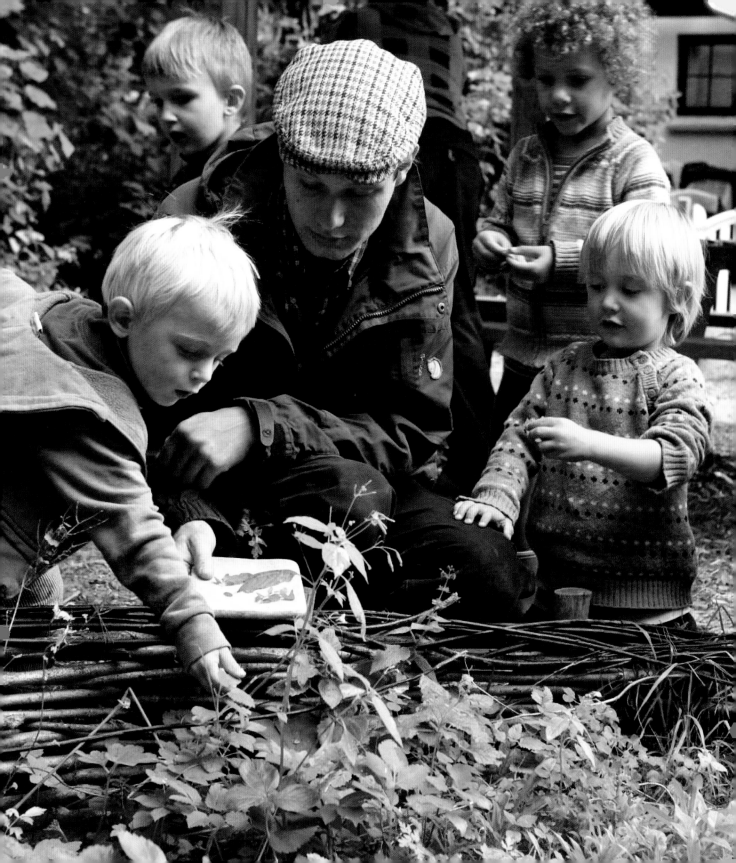

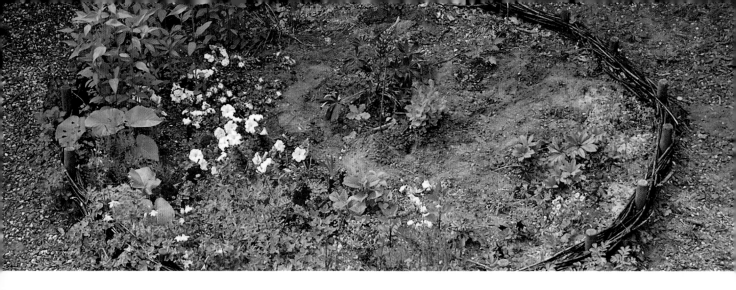

Baked plums

Makes approx. 2 l (4 US pints)
1 kg (2 lb 3 oz) plums
2 tbsp maple syrup
1 tbsp white balsamic vinegar
seeds from 1 vanilla pod
cardamom pods or cinnamon sticks
  (whichever you prefer)

1. Cut the plums in half, remove the stones and spread them out on a deep baking tray.
2. Mix all the other ingredients and drizzle over the plums.
3. Bake at 200°C (400°F) for 10–15 minutes.

You can use this in many ways. Here are some of our favourites: as a porridge topping, as a rustic jam, or in a plum trifle with macaroni and whipped cream.

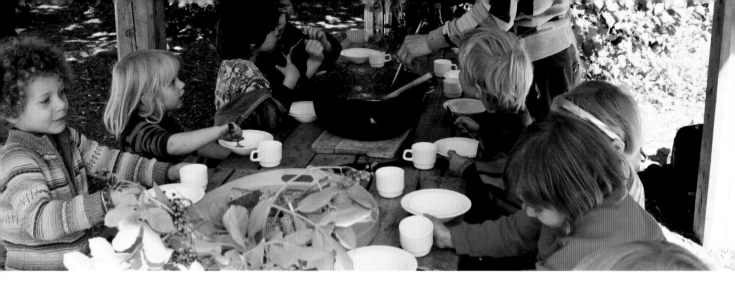

Plum relish

Makes approx. 2 l (4 US pints)
1 red onion
2 tbsp oil
½ tsp mustard seeds
½ tsp allspice
1 apple
1 tbsp cider vinegar
1 portion of baked plums (see recipe opposite)
2 cinnamon sticks
sea salt

1. Finely chop the red onion and fry in oil with the mustard seeds and allspice.
2. Finely chop the apple and add it to the pan with the vinegar.
3. Add the plums, cinnamon sticks and salt to taste.
4. Pour the relish into sterilised jars and leave to cool before sealing. Jars taken straight from the dishwasher will be sterile. Store in the fridge.

Lantern biscuits

In mid-November we celebrate the Lantern Festival, one of the most beautiful and atmospheric festivals of the year. In preparation, we paint paper lanterns, and go looking in the woods for suitable branches to tie them to. On the evening of the festival, children, teachers, parents, grandparents and anyone else who wants to take part, meet after sunset. Every child has a lantern with a tea light inside, and we walk through the woods, singing songs about light, with the bright lanterns lighting our way. In one of the songs we call on Morten, the guardian who watches over our houses at night. Eventually, Morten the Guardian appears with a sack full of lantern biscuits, which his wife has baked for the children.

Makes approx. 30 biscuits
60 g (2 oz) rye flour
55 g (2 oz) cornflour
35g sesame seeds
½ tsp herb salt or sea salt
½ tsp maple syrup
50 g (1 ¾ oz) unsalted butter or coconut butter
2–3 tbsp water

1. Mix all the dry ingredients, then add the salt and syrup.
2. Rub the butter into the mixture.
3. Knead the dough, adding a splash of water to bind it. Leave the dough to rest in the fridge for at least half an hour.
4. Roll the dough into a circle, 2 mm thick. Use a glass or cookie cutter to cut out individual biscuits.
5. Bake at 180°C (350°F) for 20 minutes.

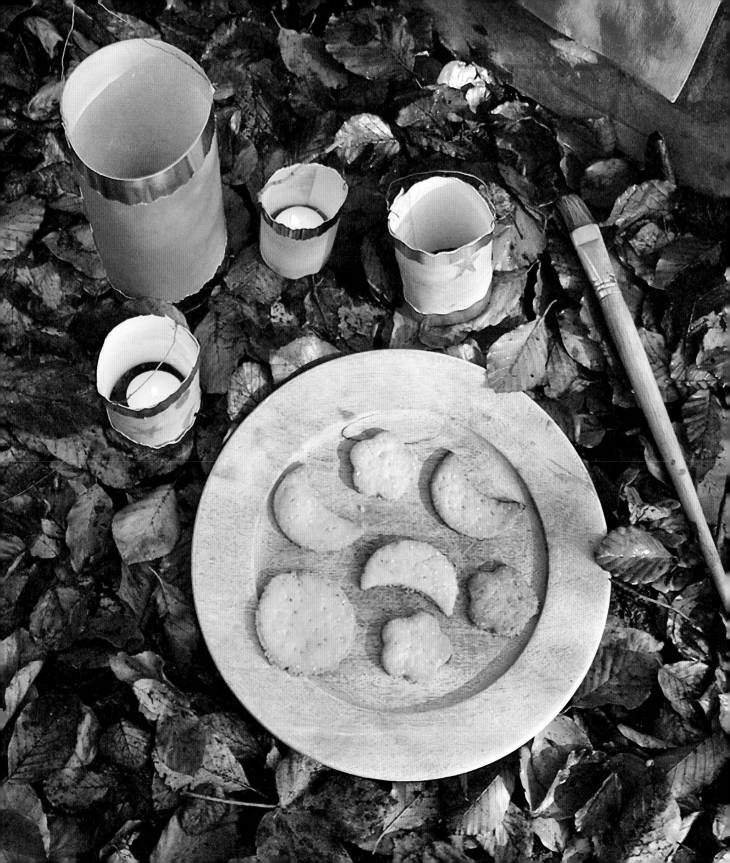

Autumnal raspberry biscuits

Makes 40 mini biscuits

Dough

150 g (5 ¼ oz) plain flour
50 g (1 ¾ oz) sifted spelt flour
1 pinch baking powder
50 g (1 ¾ oz) ground almonds (or very finely chopped almonds)
180 g (6 ⅓ oz) cold butter
3 organic egg yolks
50 g (1 ¾ oz) icing sugar

Apple compote (you will need 3–4 tbsp)

2 apples, such as Cox, sliced thinly
3 tbsp agave syrup
3 tbsp water
seeds from ¼ vanilla pod

Decoration

melted dark chocolate
apple crisps

1. Cook the ingredients for the compote until the apples are soft, then mash.
2. Mix the 2 types of flour, baking powder and ground almonds.
3. Cube the butter and rub it into the mixture.
4. Add the eggs and icing sugar.
5. Knead the dough until smooth and put it in a plastic bag. Leave it to rest in the fridge for around 2 hours.
6. Dust a worktop with some flour and roll the dough into 2 long rectangles, 3 mm (⅛ in) thick.
7. Bake at 180°C (350°F) for around 20 minutes.
8. Cut into individual biscuits.
9. Spread apple compote on a biscuit and top with another biscuit.
10. Decorate with dark chocolate and apple crisps.

The white balls in the photo are macadamia nuts, which can be used instead of almonds. There is a thin layer of compote between the biscuits.

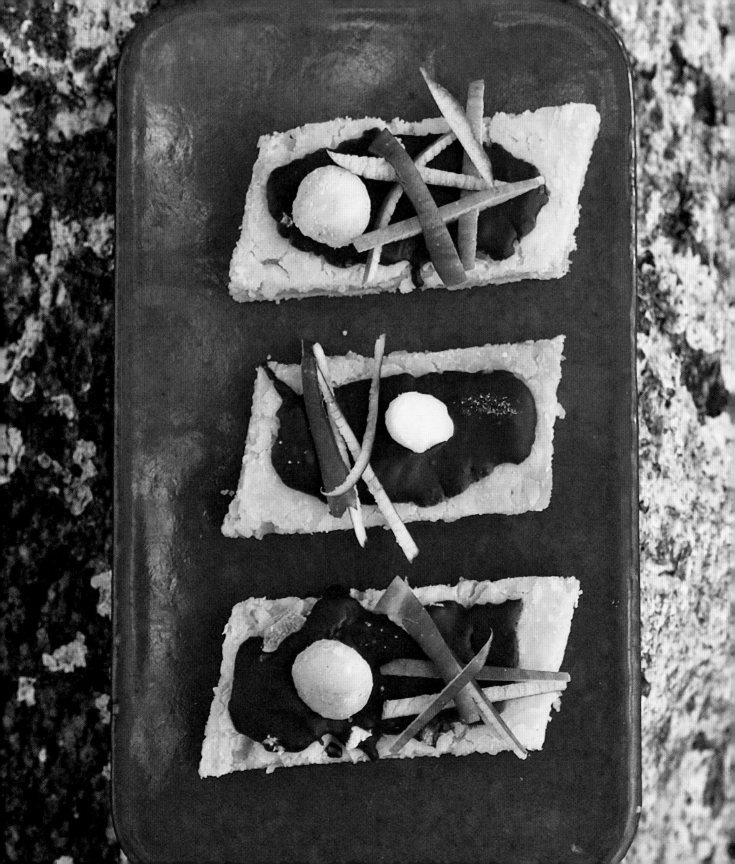

Michaelmas

At Bonsai we celebrate Saint Michael's day at the end of September, when autumn has really arrived. This festival symbolises the struggle between light and darkness, good and evil; we search for our inner courage to fight the dragon within, and this battle girds us for the cold season. In preparation for the festival we find sticks in the forest, which we whittle into mighty swords. The day before the festival we leave our swords out in the garden and the next morning it is always exciting to see if Saint Michael has sprinkled them with star dust.

On the day of the festival, the children are given blue or red capes to wear. We go into the great hall, which is lit by a big crystal mountain made of rock crystal, rose quartz, candles and little tin foil parcels full of raisins and nuts. We sit down in the semi-dark and admire the mountain while listening to the legend of Saint Michael. Then the children, one by one, walk up to the adults to be knighted. Afterwards we go outside and stamp and stomp and swing our swords to scare off every last dragon! Once the battle is over, we take our seats at the beautifully decorated long table and eat the blood-red soup Nana has made for us from amazing seasonal beetroots.

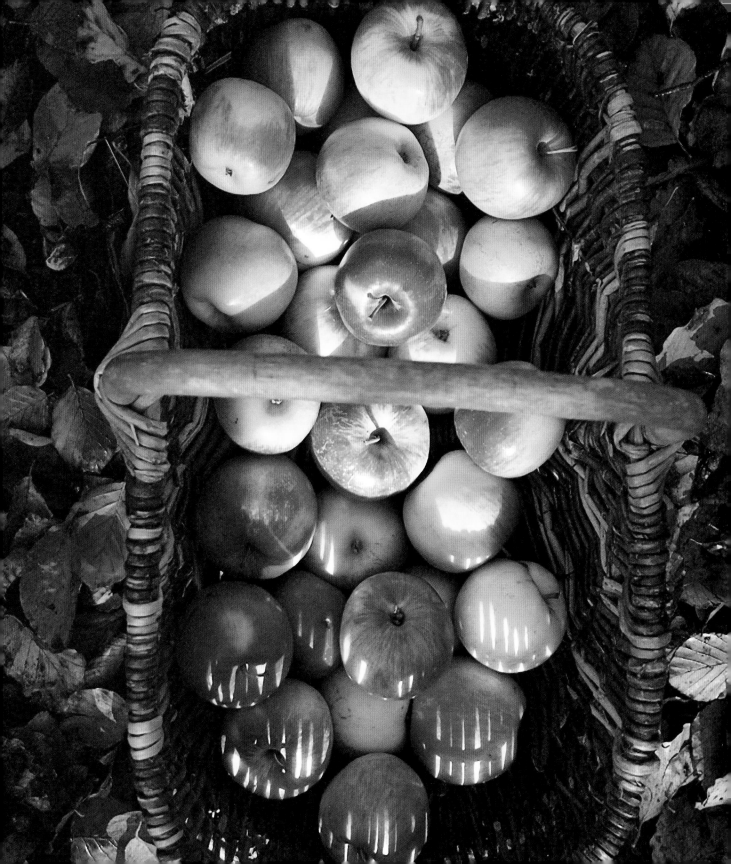

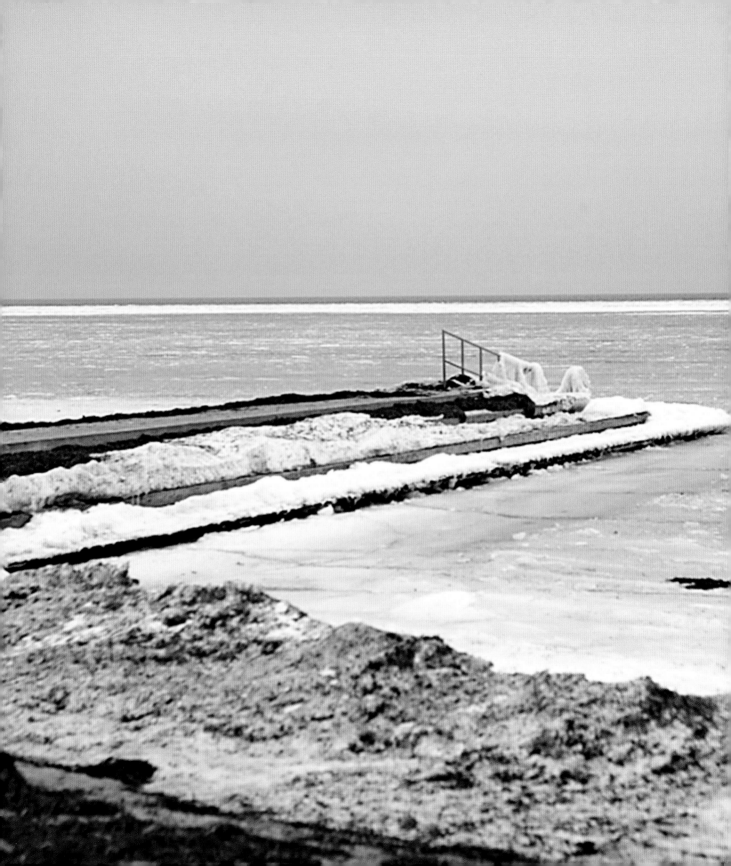

Winter

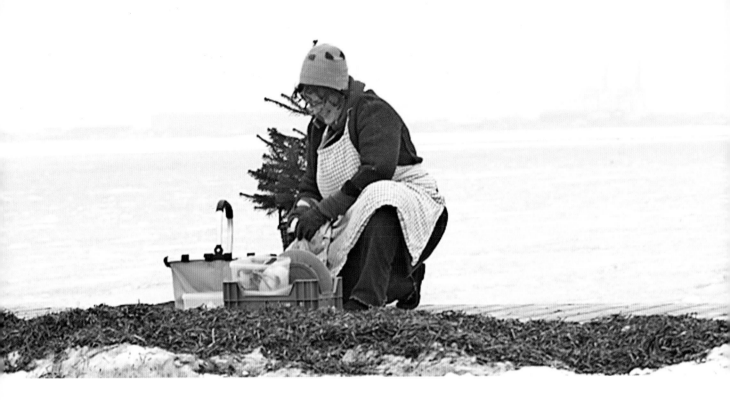

The sun rises late and sets early, but the handful of daylight hours we are given shine all the more brightly through nature's white and grey tones: the snow, the cold and the frost. The intense reds and oranges that characterise the season's beautiful sunrises contrast with the bleak winter palette and seem even more mesmerising. We are energised and empowered by what little light there is in the dark winter months.

Many adults think of winter as something they just have to get through. We associate the season with bad weather, treacherous roads and icy car windows that have to be scraped in the cold morning gloom. And there's definitely some truth in that. But it's not how children see winter. They ponder why there's no life in the forest. Where are the animals and plants? When they dig holes in the ground there are no earthworms, woodlice,

flowers or green leaves to be found. Children are experts at harnessing the peculiar qualities of winter as the elements are transformed, taking on new shapes: water turns to ice; rain becomes snow; our breath, normally invisible, comes out as 'smoke'. As long as children are dressed warmly and comfortably, they adore exploring these effects, so let them roam free.

The notion that winters are for staying indoors with a warm fire and hot soup is only partly true: we do eat a lot of soup! Winter's bounty consists primarily of large, strange tubers and the stalks and heads of giant cabbages, which are just waiting to be made into soup and served with hefty chunks of delicious homemade bread. Root vegetables are an important source of nutrients in the winter – swedes (the lemons of the north) in particular contain a lot of vitamin C – so let children work and play with root vegetables in the kitchen and outdoors. Try our recipe for wrapping root vegetables in homemade play dough and cooking them over a fire in their own juices (see p. 158). It's a fun activity for children, which will help to develop their relationship with food, and the results are excellent.

When it comes to the youngest children, up to three years old, sensory experiences such as light and sound make the biggest impression. They get excited about simple things: the rustling of leaves, birdsong and the bushy tails of squirrels. Slightly older children are tougher and want to engage more actively with nature: taste it, touch it, romp through it – so let them. But regardless of age group, it's important to bear in mind that children live in the present, they want to get the most out of every moment and they don't want to miss a thing! Following the rhythm of the seasons and being in touch with nature is part of healthy child development – and that includes winter. So we must remember to give children plenty of opportunity to play outdoors in the winter too.

Winter activities

During the winters when we're blessed with magical white snow, the opportunities for playing outdoors are endless: we can go sledging, skiing, skating or sliding, build snow caves, snowmen and snow forts, throw snowballs and make snow angels.

When nature wears white as far as the eye can see, a special feeling of peace and stillness envelops us. Sounds are muffled. When we walk through the snow, we hear a unique, crisp, creaking sound, and the feeling of compressed snow sticking to the soles of our boots grows with each step we take. The handful of animals that dare to venture out of their lairs, crossing the lawn in search of food or company, leave clearly visible paw prints in the snow – who can guess what animal that is? Maybe we can draw pictures of the tracks when we get home and make up a story about what the animal saw on its snowy journey.

This doesn't mean, of course, that only white winters can be enjoyable. On those days when nature wraps itself all in grey, it still provides endless possibilities for children to explore: there are trees to climb and there's always a branch or stone that merits closer scrutiny. Watch the sunrise on a frosty morning, or try looking up! With no leaves hiding their branches you can suddenly see the shape of the trees, their old, gnarled branches or new ones, streamlined and supple, making their way in the world.

A playground might get tedious at some point, but nature is always changing. Whatever the season, if you're going for a walk in the woods, it's a good idea to take a bag or wear a jacket with big pockets. Children love collecting stones and pebbles, weirdly twisted sticks, acorns, pretty leaves. If children carry what they pick up, they soon learn how heavy things are and that they might have to forego a thing or two. That, in turn, can help teach them to prioritise. If you collect stones, it's fun to paint them when you get back; they make good birthday presents for children's friends.

Children in nature

- Children learn through sensory experiences and movement.
- Children's imagination and sensory abilities grow in contact with nature.
- Children's motor skills improve when they move across uneven ground.
- Playing in nature strengthens children's muscles, makes them limber and improves their balance and spatial awareness.
- Outdoor activities improve children's attention spans and encourage peacefulness and creativity.
- Children who spend a lot of time outdoors are less often ill.
- When children spend a lot of time in nature, they develop a deep affection for it, which contributes to environmental awareness.

Celebrating light

The dark winter months are also a time of light and celebration. Indoors, we create the light that we are missing from the natural world, for example at Advent, the winter solstice, Christmas and New Year. No matter what our winter traditions, we usually light candles, which captivate children, as though little stories were hidden in their flickering flames – and who knows, maybe they are.

Advent at Bonsai

We start our Advent celebrations at the end of November, to spark an inner light that will guide us through the darkest time of the year. On the night before the Advent festival we arrange fresh evergreens in a large spiral and place a big church candle in the middle. We push small candles into red apples for all the children. When the children arrive in the morning, they walk into the darkened room in small groups. We then light the big candle and the children sit around the edge of the spiral watching the glow at its heart. One by one, the children are given an apple, and they walk into the spiral alone to light their candle from the big candle. They then place their candle at the edge of the spiral and go back to sit down. We sing a candle lighting song for each child, and when everyone has lit their candle we listen to a Christmas story while eating tangerines and chocolate, soaking up the glow of the candlelight.

Candle, candle burning bright,
Shining in the cold dark night.
We light a candle here today,
We light a candle for … (name of child)

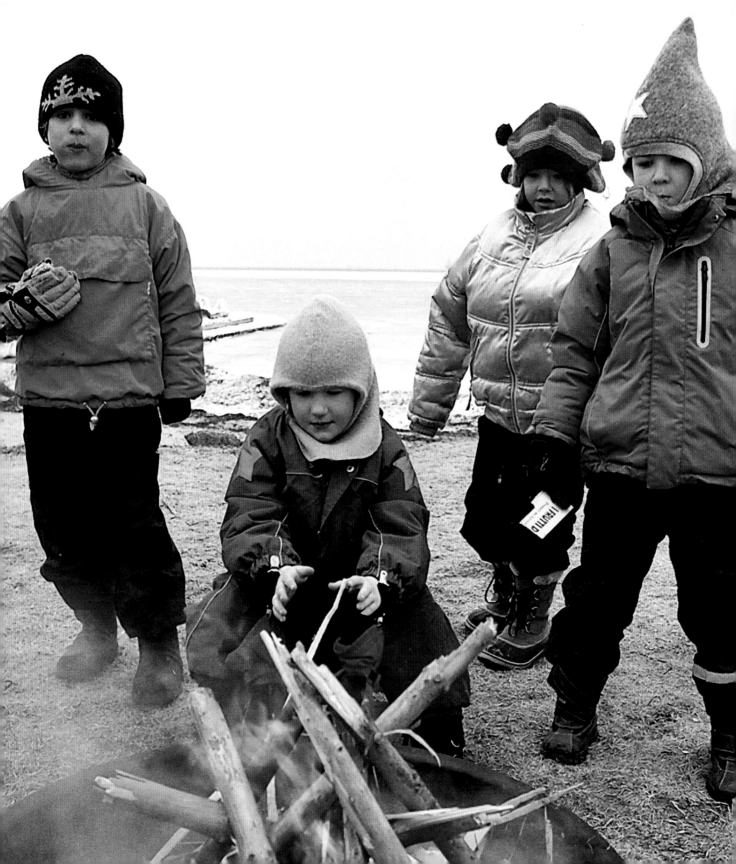

Christmas at Bonsai

Throughout December we sing carols and tell Christmas stories. We perform nativity plays every day, with songs and narration, and the children try different roles. We make paper hearts and hang them in the windows. A little house elf lives in each kindergarten room and every night, when the children have gone home, he comes out to check whether we have tidied up properly. Every day the house elf leaves little surprises for us and at lunchtime he comes in to see the children and tell them which one of them he dreamed about last night; that child then gets a little present to take home. We bake Christmas cookies with the children, and invite parents to see our nativity play and try our homemade cookies.

Fastelavn (carnival) at Bonsai

In preparation for the pre-Lent *Fastelavn* celebration, we collect birch or willow branches that we tie into bundles with the children's names on. All the bundles are hung from the ceiling with string, awaiting decorations. With their natural beauty, the bundles look pretty and festive the way they are, but children who are old enough love to make paper masks, cats or flowers out of tissue. Children enjoy their *Fastelavn* bundles more if they can design and decorate them themselves.

Every year, the kindergarten staff chooses a theme for the party's decorations and fancy dress, such as the circus, a treasure island, woodland animals, a fairy-tale ball and so on. The theme might make the *Fastelavn* party seem more rigid and less free, but in our experience, children enjoy being part of a meaningful whole, in which each component is important and everyone plays a crucial role in the big adventure.

Three weeks before the party we start singing *Fastelavn* songs and telling stories about the transformation so closely associated with *Fastelavn*. The day before the party the staff hangs little gifts on the bundles of branches and decorates the room according to that year's theme. The parents make *Fastelavn* buns (Shrovetide buns). On the day, the children arrive in costume and go straight to the main hall. The party starts with a story in which both the children and adults play different parts, such as animals, princesses or pirates. Then we eat buns. Every child gets to take their *Fastelavn* bundle home afterwards, of course. If you put the *Fastelavn* branches in water, they will sprout leaves: willow will grow downy catkins and birch will grow tender green leaves.

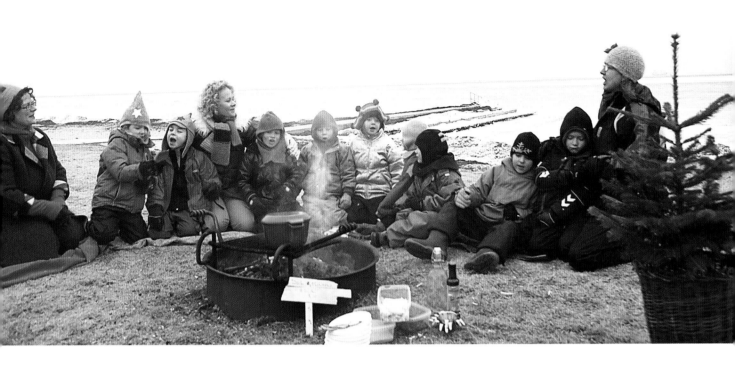

Children, adults and creativity

From a pedagogical point of view, the process followed during children's creative activities is much more important than the result. Children want to be active and equal participants in the creative process; they should be allowed to choose their own designs and set their own pace. Children will be much more proud of something they created with their own hands than of something made by their teacher or parent, and we must accept the fact that children's aesthetic sensibilities don't always correspond with our own! If activities are carefully planned and enough time is set aside, we should be able to let creative play unfold of its own accord.

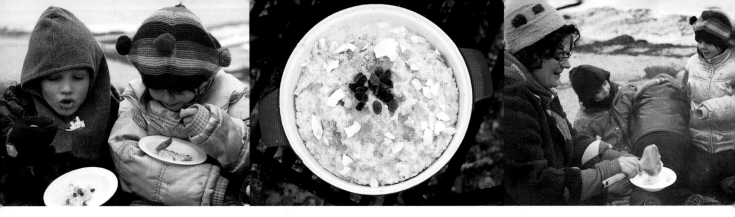

Rice pudding

This slightly healthier version of the traditional Danish rice pudding is nothing less than delicious, and the topping is highly addictive.

Serves a family of 4
250 ml (1 cup) whipping cream
250 ml (1 cup) pudding rice
100 ml (½ cup) water
1 tsp agave syrup
½ tsp herb salt
1.5 l (3 US pints) boiling water

Topping
100 g (3 ½ oz) raisins or dried fruit
toasted coconut flakes seasoned with cinnamon
flaxseed oil or thistle oil

Serves 40 children
3 l (6 ⅓ US pints) whipping cream
3 kg (6 lb 10 oz) pudding rice
5 l (10 ½ US pints) water
4 tsp agave syrup
1 tsp herb salt
3 l (6 ⅓ US pints) boiling water

Topping
700 g (1 lb 9 oz) raisins or dried fruit
toasted coconut flakes seasoned with cinnamon
flaxseed oil or thistle oil

1. Bring the cream to a boil in a bain-marie to avoid the risk of burning.
2. Pour the rice and water into a heavy pan, bring to the boil and leave to simmer for 20–30 minutes, stirring continuously.
3. Add the boiling cream, agave syrup and salt to the rice. Gradually add boiling water to the mix over the course of 10 minutes or so. Then leave on the heat until the rice is cooked.
4. Serve with dried fruit, the coconut-cinnamon mix and a drizzle of oil as an alternative to the traditional butter.

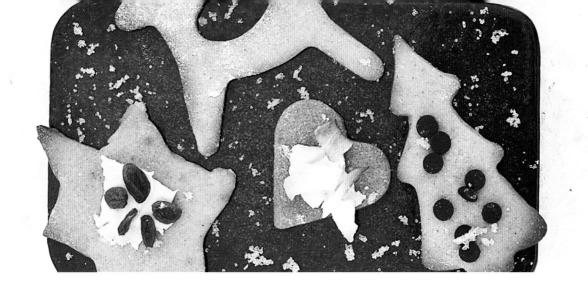

Christmas biscuits

This wonderful biscuit dough can be rolled out again and again by little hands without being ruined, and it doesn't contain raw eggs, so little bakers can safely conduct little quality controls as they go.

Makes 90–100 biscuits
100 g (3 ½ oz) butter or coconut butter
250 g (9 oz) muscovado or demerara sugar
200 ml (⅞ cup) apricot or fig puree
  (see p. 139)
1 tbsp ground cinnamon
2 tsp ground ginger
1 tbsp baking soda
300 ml (1 ¼ cups) milk or rice milk
1 kg (2 lb 3 oz) plain or spelt flour

Decoration
chocolate buttons or dried fruit and
  chopped nuts or almonds

1. Melt the butter and sugar over a low heat in a heavy pan. Remove from the heat.
2. Add the fruit purée, spices and baking soda. Slowly pour in the milk and leave to cool completely.
3. Stir in the flour, little by little, making sure the dough does not get too hard.
4. Knead the dough well, adding more flour if it gets too sticky, then refrigerate overnight.
5. Roll out the dough very thinly, no more than 7 mm (¼ inch) thick, and cut out shapes with cookie cutters. Decorate them any way you please.
6. Place the biscuits on a baking tray lined with greaseproof paper and bake at 200°C (400°F) for around 5 minutes.

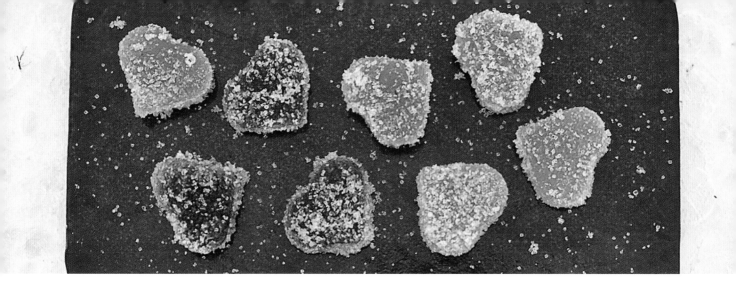

Fruit pastilles

This is an easy way to make your own natural sweeties. These homemade wine gums don't contain gelatine so they are suitable for vegetarians and vegans.

Makes approx. 40 sweets
500 ml (1 US pint) cordial, preferably organic
1 tbsp lemon juice
2 tbsp agave syrup
1 tsp agar flakes
demerara sugar

1. Mix the cordial, lemon juice and syrup and bring to the boil.
2. Remove from the heat and beat in the agar flakes.
3. Pour the mixture into a glass or porcelain dish, measuring approx. 20 cm (8 in) square. Leave to set in the fridge for a few hours or overnight.
4. When set, cut into shapes and roll in demerara sugar.

Apricot or fig purée

100 g (3½ oz) dried apricots or figs
300 ml (1¼ cups) water

1. Soak the fruit in water for 2 hours.
2. Then boil it in fresh water until completely soft.
3. Allow it to cool a little, then blend to a smooth purée.

. . . .

Swede muffins

These muffins are a treat for our youngest children, who usually prefer bread and buns to cake. For a larger batch, simply double the recipe.

Makes 10 muffins

500 g (1 lb 2 oz) quinoa
300 g (10 ½ oz) swede
1 tsp thyme
1 clove of garlic
1 pinch herb salt
200 ml (⅞ cup) water

2 organic eggs
2 tbsp plain flour
100 g (3 ½ oz) finely diced tofu

Decoration
finely diced tofu (optional)

1. Cook the quinoa according to the instructions on the box and drain any remaining water.
2. Grate the swede coarsely and mix it with the quinoa and remaining ingredients to a nice, smooth dough.
3. Divide the dough into 10 muffin cases and sprinkle some tofu on top.
4. Bake at 180°C (350°F) for at least 40 minutes.

Swede ragout

The swede is one of northern Europe's most wonderful, but often forgotten, root vegetables. It is packed full of vitamin C, which can help keep winter colds at bay.

1 swede
2 red onions
½ red pepper
150 g (5 ¼ oz) fresh broad beans or
   blanched kale
2 tbsp oil for frying
1 clove of garlic
20 g (¾ oz) ginger
1 tsp herb salt
freshly ground pepper
lemon juice (optional)

5 swedes
8 red onions
2 red peppers
800 g (1 lb 12 oz) fresh broad beans or
   blanched kale
100 ml (½ cup) oil for frying
4 cloves of garlic
75 g (2 ⅔ oz) ginger
3 tsp herb salt
freshly ground pepper
lemon juice (optional)

1. Start by preparing the vegetables. Peel and dice the swede. Dice the onions and peppers. Halve the broad beans lengthwise.
2. Heat the oil in a heavy pan and sweat the swede and onion. Before they're completely soft, add the pepper and beans.
3. Leave to simmer for 10 minutes, then season with garlic, ginger, salt, pepper and lemon juice, if using.

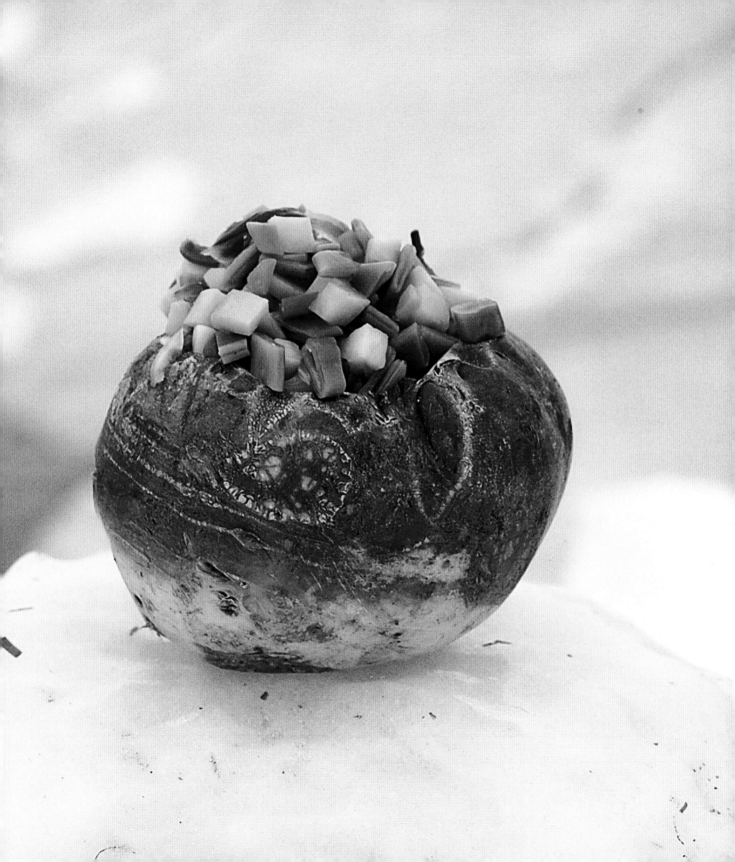

Beetroot (beet) soup with kale and beans

This blood-red soup with jet-black beans should be served alongside a really scary story!

Serves a family of 4
1 onion, chopped
1 potato, peeled and diced
2 cloves of garlic, chopped
3 large beetroots (beets), peeled and diced
1 parsnip or celery stick, peeled and diced
1 l (2 US pints) water
pinch of herb salt or sea salt
freshly ground pepper

Topping
150 g (5 ¼ oz) black beans (pre-soaked for
   24 hours)
80 g (2 ¾ oz) kale, blanched
1 large red onion, chopped
1 tbsp olive oil
2 tbsp white balsamic vinegar
1 tsp herb salt or sea salt
1 tbsp honey
juice and zest of 1 organic lemon

Serves 40 children
10 onions, chopped
5 kg (11 lb) potatoes, peeled and diced
9 cloves of garlic, chopped
3 kg (6 lb 10 oz) beetroot (beets), peeled and diced
1 kg (2 lb 3 oz) celeriac, peeled and diced
10 l (21 US pints) water
1 tbsp herb salt or sea salt
freshly ground pepper

Topping
1.5 kg (3 lb 5 oz) black beans (pre-soaked for
   24 hours)
1 kg (2 lb 3 oz) kale, blanched
5 red onions, chopped
100 ml (½ cup) olive oil
3 tbsp white balsamic vinegar
2 tbsp herb salt or sea salt
3 tbsp honey
juice and zest of 4 organic lemons

Topping

1. Cook the pre-soaked black beans in plenty of water until soft (around 45 minutes).
2. Chop the kale and mix with the beans.
3. Sweat the onion in oil without letting it brown.
4. Add the vinegar, salt and honey. Mix in the beans and kale.
5. If you like, flavour with lemon juice and zest and add an extra dash of oil.

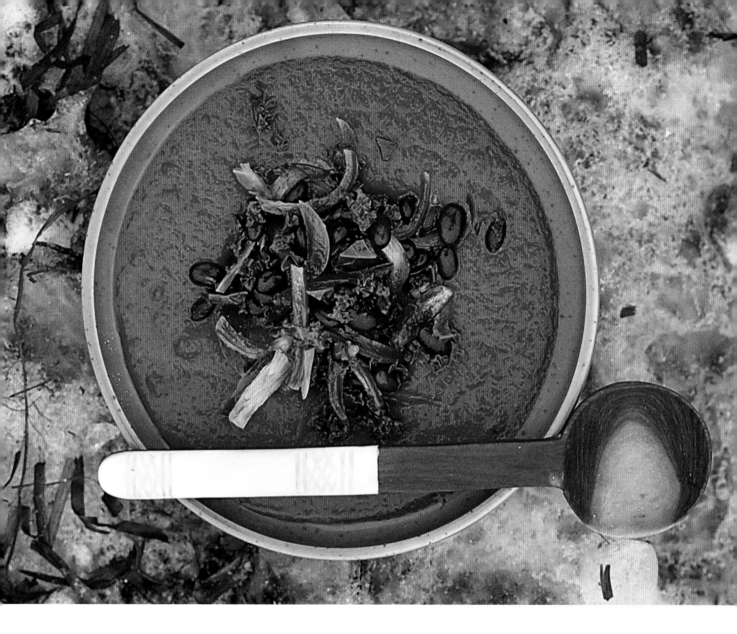

Soup

1. Start by frying the onion, potato and garlic in a dash of oil until they start to soften, then add the beetroot and celeriac (celery or parsnip).
2. Pour in the water and leave to cook for 30 minutes.
3. Blend and season with salt and pepper to taste.
4. Serve the soup hot with a helping of the nutritious topping.

Beetroot (beet) bread with seaweed

This luscious pink bread with seaweed adds much-needed nutrients to tired winter bodies, young and old. If you don't have time to prove the dough cold, you can add another 25 g (1 oz) yeast and prove for 50 minutes before following the baking instructions below.

Makes 2 loaves

25 g (1 oz) fresh yeast
750 ml (1 ½ US pints) lukewarm water
2 tbsp salt
4 tbsp honey
125 g (4 ½ oz) arame seaweed
3 coarsely grated beetroots (beets)
75 ml (⅓ cup) oil
125 g (4 ½ oz) cracked wheat
approx. 750 g (1 lb 10 oz) plain or spelt flour

1. Dissolve the yeast in the water and stir in the salt and honey. Add the remaining ingredients and knead well.
2. Leave the dough to prove overnight in the fridge.
3. Take the dough out and split it into 2 equal sections. Knead each briefly and place on baking trays lined with greaseproof paper.
4. Leave to prove a second time for 30 minutes.
5. Bake the bread at 180°C (350°F) for around 45 minutes.

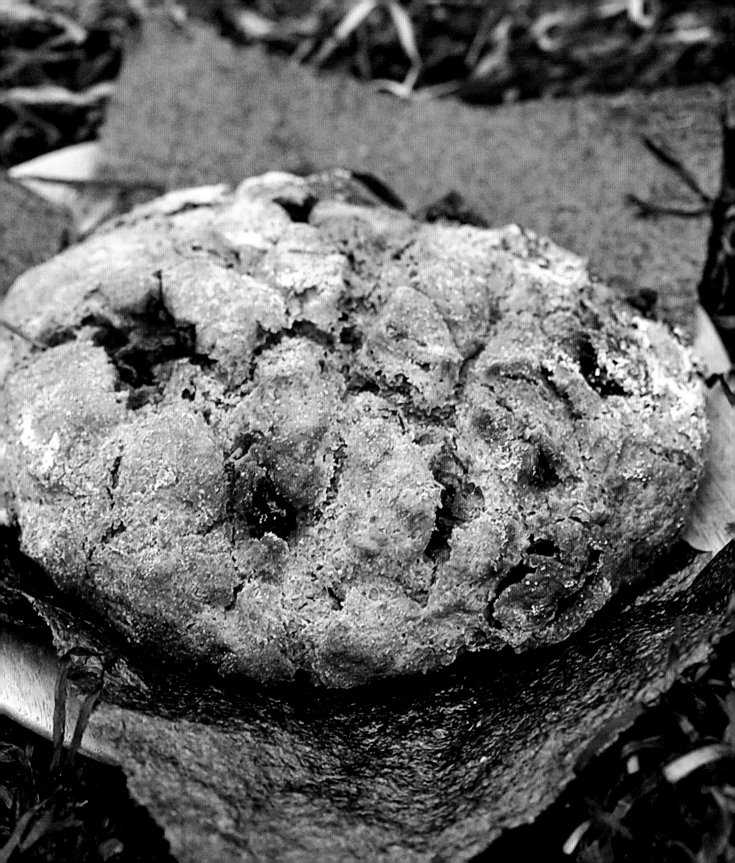

Beetroot (beet) sandwich spread

This spread tastes great on rye bread or as a sandwich filling. It keeps for up to a week in the fridge and freezes well, so even if you have a small family it's a good idea to make a big batch.

Serves a family of 4
500 g (1 lb 2 oz) white beans
1 medium-sized beetroot (beet)
1 tsp herb salt
2 cloves of garlic, finely chopped
2 tbsp tahini
1 tbsp white balsamic vinegar
5 tbsp oil
200–300 ml (1–1 ¼ cups) boiling water

Serves 40 children
3 kg (6 lb 10 oz) white beans
1 kg (2 lb 3 oz) beetroot (beet)
1 tbsp herb salt
8 cloves of garlic, finely chopped
1 jar of tahini
100 ml (½ cup) white balsamic vinegar
200–300 ml (1–1 ¼ cups) oil
2–3 l (4–6 US pints) boiling water

1. Pre-soak the beans in water overnight.
2. Cook in fresh water until soft (around 45 minutes).
3. Peel and grate the beetroot (beet).
4. Mix all the ingredients, except the water, in a bowl. Add water to achieve a good consistency.
5. Season the spread and put it in a dish or bowl. Cover and refrigerate.

White-on-white winter quiche

Food for children is often brightly coloured, so it can be both fun and challenging to create a meal using just one colour, for example a white winter or spring green meal. This pie can be served as a starter or a main course.

Makes 1 quiche

Pastry	Filling	Custard
175 g (6 oz) spelt flour	150 g (5 ¼ oz) Jerusalem artichoke	3 organic eggs
125 g (4 ½ oz) butter	100 g (3 ½ oz) swede	3 tbsp milk or organic coconut milk
3 tbsp water	50 g (1 ¾ oz) almonds or pistachio nuts	1 tsp sea salt
½ tsp herb salt		freshly ground pepper

1. Start by making the pastry: rub the butter into the flour and salt. Bind the dough together with water, and leave to cool in the fridge.
2. Wash and finely slice the artichokes and peel and finely slice the swede. Chop the nuts, unless you bought them chopped.
3. Mix the ingredients for the custard.
4. Take the pastry out of the fridge. If it's too hard to work with, leave it on the kitchen table for 20 minutes until it feels more pliable. Roll it into a round shape, roughly 7 mm (¼ in) thick.
5. Lay your pastry over a buttered flan dish, pushing the pastry carefully into the corners.
6. Put the filling into the pastry case and pour over the custard.
7. Bake at 200°C (400°F) for 45 minutes.

Lovable Brussels sprouts

You may think I've lost my mind trying to feed Brussels sprouts to young children. But I think I've achieved the impossible with this recipe. It's very satisfying to see even the youngest children wolf down sprouts!

Serves a family of 4
200 g (7 oz) Brussels sprouts
½ pomegranate
1 large organic orange

Dressing
4 tbsp olive oil
2 tbsp white balsamic vinegar
1 pinch of sea salt

Serves 40 children
2 kg (4 lb 7 oz) Brussels sprouts
2 pomegranates
5 organic oranges

Dressing
250 ml (1 cup) olive oil
100 ml (½ cup) white balsamic vinegar
1 tsp sea salt

1. Prepare the sprouts and cut them into quarters.
2. Cook them in lightly salted water until they are al dente (still slightly firm). Plunge them into cold water immediately to retain their green colour.
3. Deseed the pomegranate. Dice or segment the orange. Mix both with the sprouts.
4. Mix the ingredients for the dressing and drizzle over the salad.

• •

Brussels sprouts with sesame seeds and tamari

Serves a family of 4
300 g (10 ½ oz) Brussels sprouts
2–3 tbsp tamari or soy sauce
1 tbsp sesame seeds
1 tbsp thistle oil

Serves 40 children
4 kg (8lb 13 oz) Brussels sprouts
200 ml (⅞ cup) tamari or soy sauce
70 g (2 ½ oz) sesame seeds
100 ml (½ cup) thistle oil

1. Prepare the Brussels sprouts and boil them for around 5 minutes, depending on size.
2. Drain and toss with the tamari, oil and sesame seeds. Serve immediately.

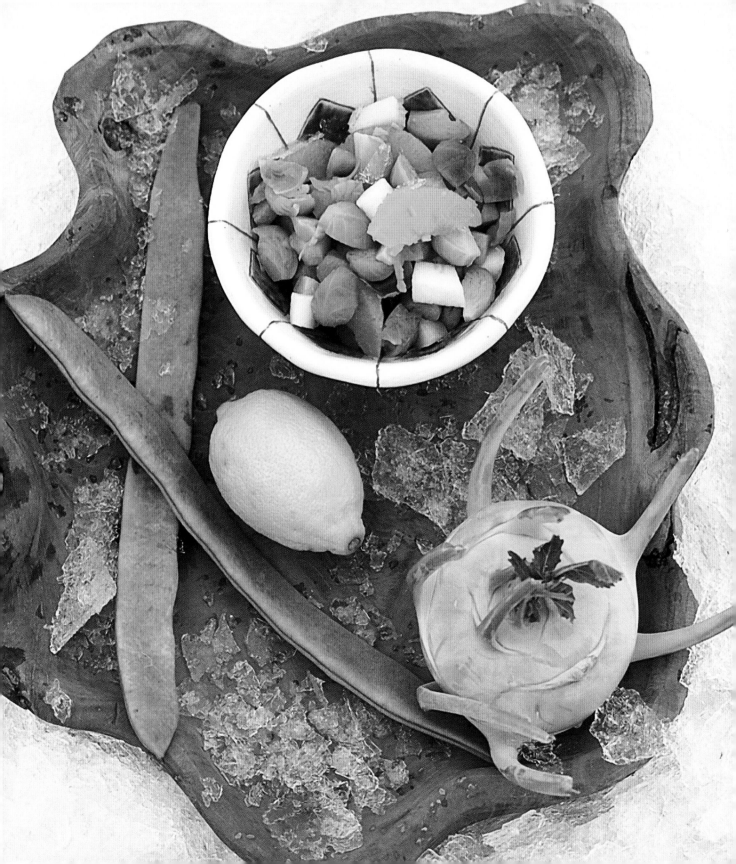

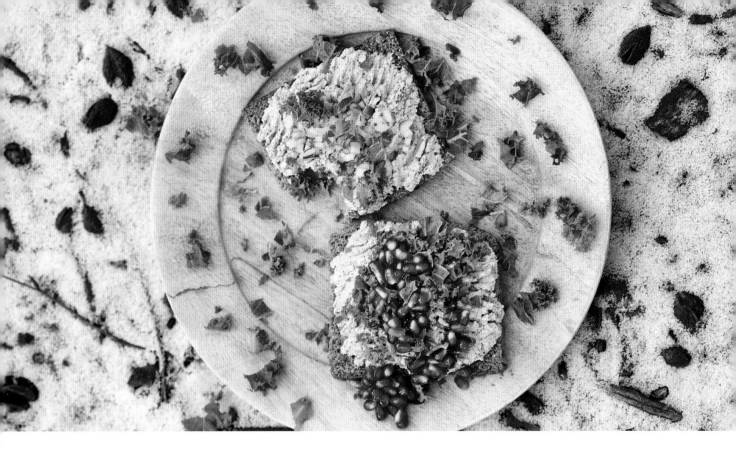

Crazy about kale!

Kale is an incredibly beautiful and flavoursome vegetable, with many possible uses. Peak season in northern Europe is winter, and it's full of vitamins C and K, which are especially important during the cold winter months.

During my restaurant days we often blanched kale to soften it and enhance its rich flavour, and served it with high-quality olive oil and pecorino.

To blanch kale, remove the leaves from the stalk; put the leaves in lightly salted boiling water and cook for 1 minute; drain and immediately plunge the leaves into ice-cold water; finally, use your hands to wring the leaves dry.

On the following pages I've included a few kale recipes that I keep coming back to.

Kale sandwich spread

Mix finely chopped, blanched kale with organic cream cheese. Season with a little garlic, herbs, salt and pepper, and you have a delicious spread to enjoy on a slice of toasted rye bread.

• •

Kale pâté

This pâté is perfect to serve for breakfast, as a starter or main course.

Serves a family of 4
100 g (3½ oz) blanched kale
1 onion
4 potatoes
juice and zest of 1 organic orange
5 organic eggs
3 tbsp water from blanching
herb salt or sea salt
freshly ground black pepper

Serves 40 children
4 kg (8lb 13 oz) blanched kale
5 onions
18 potatoes
juice and zest of 4 organic oranges
30 large, organic eggs
150 ml (⅔ cup) water from blanching
herb salt or sea salt
freshly ground black pepper

1. Finely chop the blanched kale and onion. Peel and grate the potatoes.
2. Mix the kale, onion and potato well and add the orange juice and zest.
3. Beat the eggs and blanching water together with a whisk, season with salt and pepper, and fold into the vegetable mix.
4. Grease a 8 x 25 cm (3 x 10 in) bread tin and pour in the mixture.
5. Bake the pâté at 180°C (350°F) for around 30 minutes. Test with a skewer: the pâté is ready when the skewer comes out clean.

Malfatti with kale

I learnt how to make this lovely Italian dish from Pina, my Italian 'mother', who I stayed with when I worked in Montevarchi in Italy. It's an easy dish to make for a large group of people; just put the batter in a piping bag and cut the malfatti straight into boiling water with scissors.

Serves a family of 4
150 g (5 ¼ oz) ricotta cheese
3 organic egg yolks
150 g (5 ¼ oz) plain flour
180 g (6 ⅓ oz) blanched kale, finely chopped
4 tbsp unsalted butter
1 tsp herb salt
½ tsp grated nutmeg

Serves 40 children
750 g (1 lb 10 oz) ricotta cheese
15 organic egg yolks
300 g (10 ½ oz) plain flour
3.5 kg (7 lb 11 oz) blanched kale, finely chopped
15 tbsp unsalted butter
2 tbsp herb salt
1 tsp grated nutmeg

1. Push the ricotta through a sieve.
2. Add the egg yolks and flour and stir, then add the finely chopped kale, butter and spices.
3. Bring a pan (or pans) of lightly salted water or stock to the boil.
4. Put the malfatti batter into a piping bag with a large opening, then squeeze it out, using scissors to cut individual pieces of about 2.4 cm (1 in). Leave to simmer until the malfatti float to the top.
5. Carefully remove the malfatti with a slotted spoon and leave to drain on kitchen towel or a cooling rack.
6. Serve with tomato sauce and grated Parmesan cheese.

Kale pesto

The kindergarten version of this recipe has been adjusted to suit our budget, by using almonds and sunflower seeds, which are rich in selenium, instead of pine nuts.

Serves a family of 4
200 g (7 oz) blanched kale
100 g (3 ½ oz) pine nuts
80 g (2 ¾ oz) Parmesan cheese
½ tsp sea salt
1 clove of garlic
½ tsp organic orange zest
250 ml (1 cup) quality olive oil

Serves 40 children
850 g (1 lb 14 oz) blanched kale
120 g (4 ¼ oz) sunflower seeds
200 g (7 oz) almonds, whole
250 g (9 oz) Parmesan cheese
3 tsp sea salt
5 cloves of garlic
2 tsp organic orange zest
400 ml (1 ⅔ cups) quality olive oil
200 ml (⅞ cup) boiled water (use the kale blanching water)

1. Put all the ingredients into a blender. Remember to cut the Parmesan into smaller pieces, and don't use all of the oil straight away.
2. Blend the pesto until you achieve the right consistency, and season with sea salt.

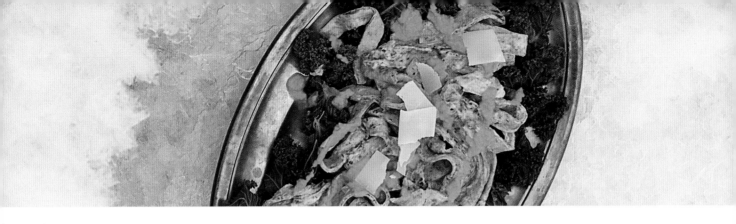

Pasta with kale

Your children will love making this pasta dish with you; it's a great challenge for little fingers on a cold winter's day. You don't need a pasta machine to roll out the dough.

Serves a family of 4
200 g (7 oz) flour ('00' grade pasta flour)
100 g (3 ½ oz) plain flour
3 organic eggs, lightly beaten
1 tbsp olive oil
75 g (2 ⅔ oz) blanched kale, finely chopped
80 g (2 ¾ oz) carrots, mashed
herb salt
freshly ground black pepper

Serves 40 children
2 kg (4 lb 7 oz) flour ('00' grade pasta flour)
1 kg (2 lb 3 oz) plain flour
16 organic eggs, lightly beaten
300 ml (1 ¼ cups) olive oil
850 g (1 lb 14 oz) blanched kale, finely chopped
1 kg (2 lb 3 oz) carrots, mashed
4 tsp herb salt
freshly ground black pepper

1. Pour the flour onto the work surface and make a well in the middle for the eggs and oil. Mix gently and start kneading the dough.
2. Add the mashed carrots, kale, salt and pepper and knead well, adding flour if necessary. The dough should be drier and firmer than typical bread dough.
3. Put the dough in a plastic bag and leave it to rest in the fridge for an hour.
4. Roll it roughly ½ cm (¼ in) thick using a pasta machine or a rolling pin and cut into strips.
5. Hang the strips over a broom handle or a thick piece of string for 1–2 hours.
6. Boil in lightly salted water for around 3–5 minutes, depending on thickness. The pasta should be al dente (with a bit of bite).

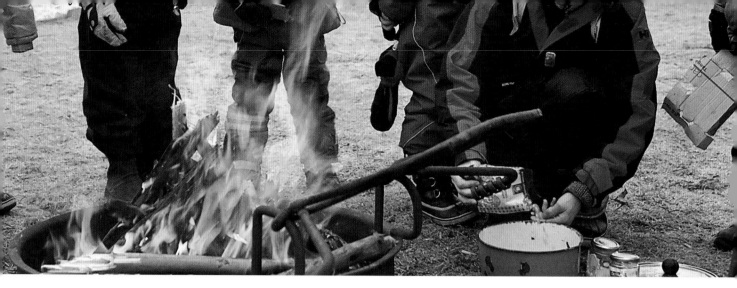

Nut pesto

This is a Nordic version of the pine nut pesto I used to make when I lived in Italy. The fat in the nuts is a valuable and necessary component in the children's diet.

Serves a family of 4
100 g (3 ½ oz) almonds, whole
100 g (3 ½ oz) hazelnuts, flaked
50 g (1 ¾ oz) walnuts
2 tbsp parsley, finely chopped
1 clove of garlic
1 tsp lovage, finely chopped
1 tsp organic orange zest
100 ml (½ cup) quality rapeseed (canola) oil
1 tsp sea salt

Serves 40 children
1 kg (2 lb 3 oz) almonds, whole
250 g (9 oz) hazelnuts, flaked
200 g (7 oz) sunflower seeds
1 bunch of parsley
4 cloves of garlic
2 tbsp lovage, finely chopped
1 tbsp organic orange zest
600–700 ml (1 ¼–1 ½ US pints) quality
   rapeseed (canola) oil
5 tsp sea salt

1. Roast each type of nut separately in a frying pan or in the oven to bring out the flavours.
2. Pulse the almonds and walnuts in a blender.
3. Mix the nut paste and flaked hazelnuts or sunflower seeds with finely chopped herbs and oil. Add garlic, orange zest and salt to taste.
4. This can be used as a pesto, a sandwich spread or a relish.

155

Nut bake

Traditional Christmas food can be a bit dull for vegetarians, but this delicious classic will light up your festive meal.

Serves 6
250 g (9 oz) celeriac
200 g (7 oz) sweet potato
350 g (12 1/3 oz) white mushrooms
100 g (3 1/2 oz) onion
100 g (3 1/2 oz) hazelnuts
100 g (3 1/2 oz) walnuts
3 tbsp tamari
freshly ground black pepper
1 tbsp sea salt
150 g (5 1/4 oz) local eating apples
100 g (3 1/2 oz) pitted prunes
2 sprigs of thyme

Serves 40 children
3 kg (6 lb 10 oz) celeriac
2.5 kg (5 lb 8 oz) sweet potato
2 kg (4 lb 7 oz) white mushrooms
1 kg (2 lb 3 oz) onions
500 g (1 lb 2 oz) hazelnuts
500 g (1 lb 2 oz) walnuts
3 tbsp tamari
freshly ground black pepper
3 tbsp sea salt
650 g (1 lb 7 oz) local eating apples
500 g (1 lb 2 oz) pitted prunes
1 bunch of thyme

1. Peel, chop and boil the celeriac and sweet potato, then mash with 100 ml (1/2 cup) of the leftover cooking water.
2. Chop or blend the nuts finely, grate the onions coarsely and chop the mushrooms. Slice the apples and halve the prunes.
3. Mix the mashed vegetables with the nuts, mushrooms, onion, herbs and seasoning to make a hash.
4. Put half of the hash in a buttered pie dish. Top with apple slices and prunes then add the rest of the hash.
5. Bake at 200°C (400°F) for around 45 minutes.
6. Serve with raw kale or white cabbage.

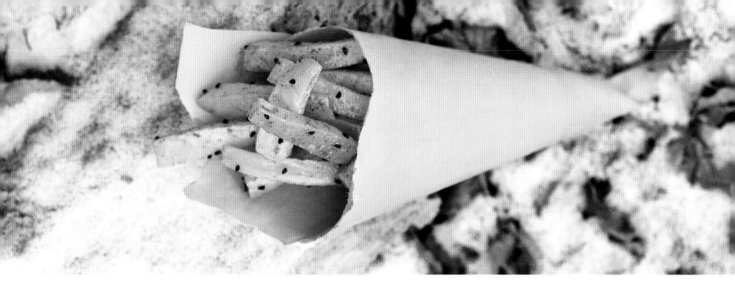

Swede fries

Serves a family of 4	Serves 40 children
1 small swede	7 swedes
2 tbsp olive oil	150 ml (⅔ cup) olive oil
1 tsp curry powder	2 tbsp curry powder
1 tsp sea salt	3 tsp sea salt
1 tsp white balsamic vinegar	3 tsp white balsamic vinegar

1. Clean and peel the swede and cut it into French fry-sized strips.
2. Use the remaining ingredients to make a dressing and toss with the fries.
3. Bake the fries on greaseproof paper at 200°C (400°F) for around 30 minutes.

Root vegetables in salt dough

You can use celeriac, swede, beetroot (beet), potato, sweet potato, Jerusalem artichoke, carrot or parsnip.

Serves a family of 4
130 g (4 ½ oz) plain flour
100 g (3 ½ oz) salt
3 tbsp water

Serves 40 children
1 kg (2 lb 3 oz) plain flour
500 g (1 lb 2 oz) salt
500–600 ml (1–1 ¼ US pints) water

1. Make the dough and leave it to rest in the fridge for 30 minutes.
2. Wrap whole root vegetables in the dough and bake at 200°C (400°F). Note that the cooking time varies according to the size of the vegetable.
3. Put the baked roots on the dining table and let the children peel off the dough and dig out tasty mouthfuls with teaspoons. These are delicious served with a herb butter.

Note: the dough is not for eating!

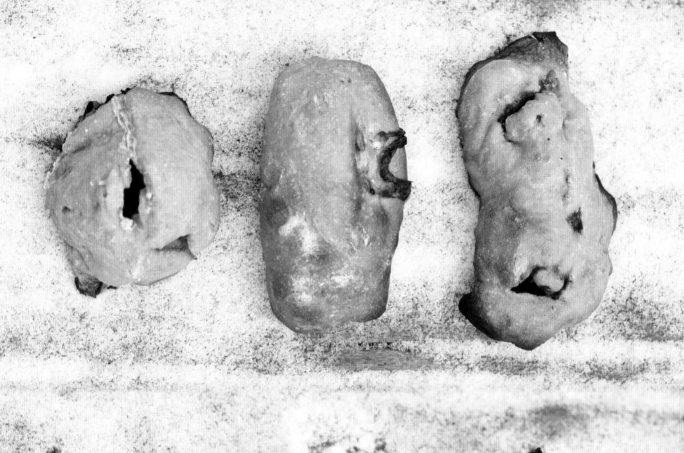

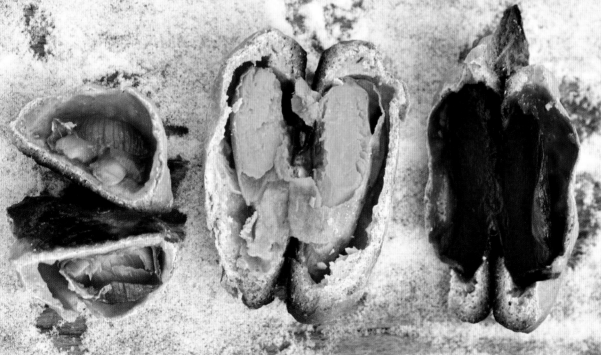

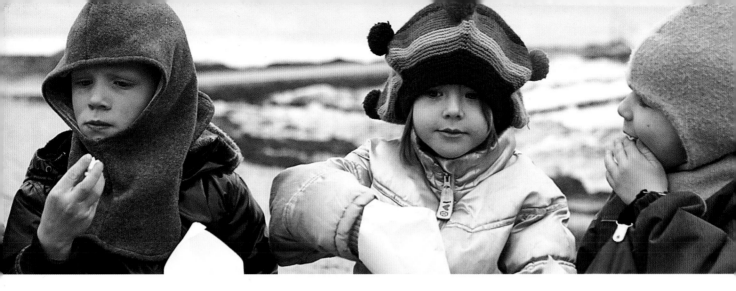

Nori crisps

Seaweed crisps taste particularly great in winter because of all the minerals they contain, and they're fun to make together too. My children love them!

Serves a family of 4
2 sheets of nori seaweed
1 tbsp rice wine vinegar
2 tbsp thistle oil
1 pinch of sea salt

1. Mix the oil, vinegar and salt to make a dressing, and use it to brush both sides of the seaweed.
2. Roast the nori in the oven at 200°C (400°F), or over the gas hob, for 2 minutes.
3. Use scissors to cut the sheets into crisps.

Tip: these seaweed crisps can also be cooked over an open fire, using skewers. Roast the seaweed until it changes colour to maximise the flavour.

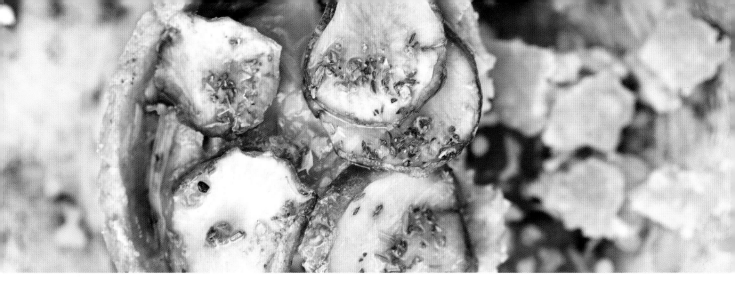

Jerusalem artichoke crisps

Adjust the number of artichokes to the size of the group you're cooking for – roughly 2 per person.

Jerusalem artichokes
1 tsp herb salt or sea salt
white balsamic vinegar
oil (use 3 parts oil to 1 part vinegar)

1. Clean the artichokes well with a sponge. It's important to leave them unpeeled because the peel helps maintain their slightly chewy consistency. Slice them thinly with a very sharp knife or a mandolin.
2. Spread the crisps out on a baking tray lined with greaseproof paper, drizzle with dressing and sprinkle with salt.
3. Bake the crisps at 200°C (400°F) for 5–7 minutes.

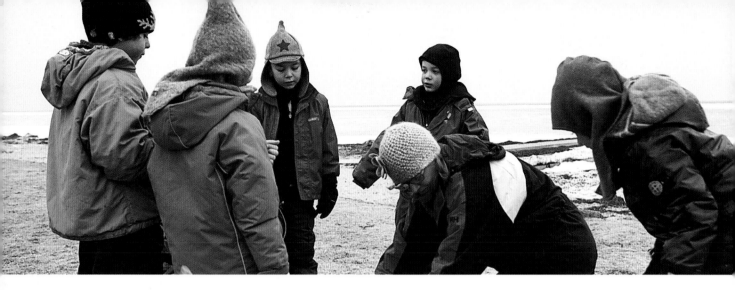

Mulled wine for children

Hot squash is lovely in the cold season and doesn't stimulate mucus production as much as hot chocolate. We serve this tasty, vitamin C-rich beverage at our lantern festival.

Serves a family of 4
200 ml (⅞ cup) concentrated elderberry cordial (or other type of cordial)
400 ml (1 ⅔ cups) water
1 organic orange
½ pomegranate

Serves 40 children
2 l (4 ¼ US pints) concentrated elderberry cordial (or other type of cordial)
3 l (6 ⅓ US pints) water
6 organic oranges
2 pomegranates

1. Bring the water to the boil and mix with the cordial.
2. Add pomegranate seeds and slices of orange for a festive look.

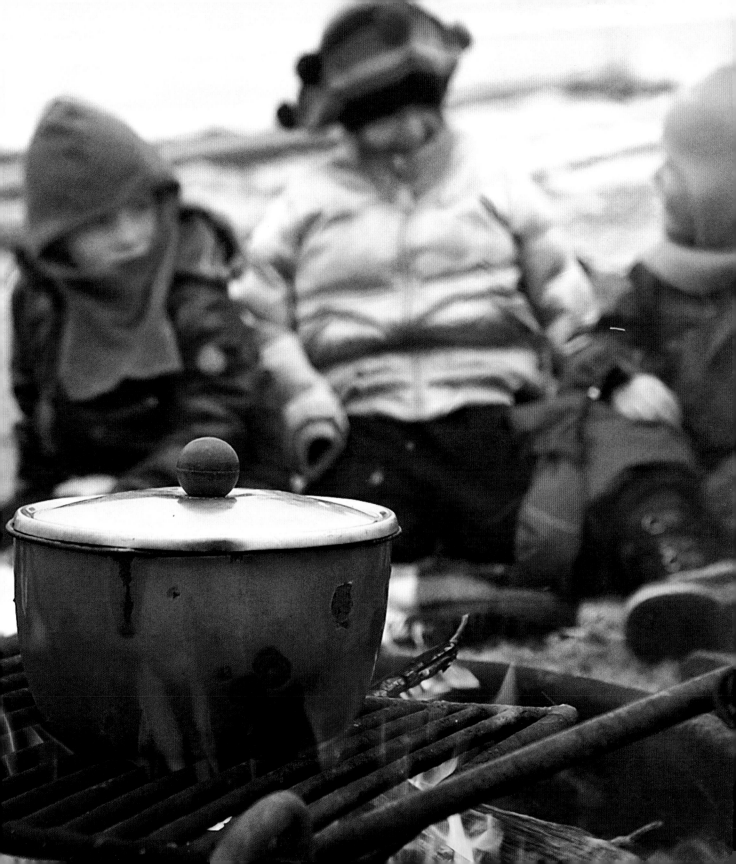

Index

millet
    Tomato and millet tabbouleh 66
mint
    Green pea cake 82
    Strawberry vinaigrette with
      pumpernickel 78
mushrooms 90
    Mushroom pâté 116
    Mushroom soup 118
    Nut bake 156
    Preserved autumn mushrooms 114

nuts
    —, almonds
      Kale pesto 153
      Nut pesto 155
      Spring tartlets 38
      White-on-white winter quiche
        147
    ——, ground almonds
      Autumnal raspberry biscuits 124
    —, Brazil
      Spinach pesto 50
    — hazelnuts
      Cured cabbage 108
      Nut bake 156
      Nut pesto 155
    —, pine
      Kale pesto 153
      Turnip carpaccio 32
    —, pistachio
      White-on-white winter quiche 147
    — walnuts
      Nut bake 156
      Nut pesto 155

parsley
    Nut pesto 155
    Spring tartlets 38
    Tomato and millet tabbouleh 66
parsnip
    Root vegetables in salt dough 158
pasta
    Green pea minestrone 83
    Malfatti with kale 152

    Pasta with kale 154
    Spinach lasagne 51
pâté
    Asparagus pâté 37
    Kale pâté 151
    Mushroom pâté 116
peanut butter
    Carrots with satay sauce 48
peanuts
    Pom's Asian bean salad 96
pear
    Cured cabbage 108
peas
    Green pea cake 82
    Green pea minestrone 83
    Green pea sandwich spread 84
pesto
    Kale pesto 153
    Nut pesto 155
    Spinach pesto 50
pickling
    Pickled cucumbers 86
    Pickled squash 98
    Preserved autumn mushrooms 114
pizza
    Potato pizza 70
plums
    Baked plums 120
    Plum relish 121
pomegranate
    Lovable Brussels sprouts 148
    Turnip carpaccio 32
porridge
    Crispbread 42
potato
    Jesper's campfire soup 112
    Root vegetables in salt dough 158
    —, new
      Green pea minestrone 83
      Potato balls 73
      Potato pizza 70
      Warm potato salad 72
    —, sweet
      Jesper's campfire soup 112
      Mild pumpkin curry 102

    Nut bake 156
    Root vegetables in salt dough 158
pumpernickel
    Strawberry vinaigrette with
      pumpernickel 78
pumpkin
    Mild pumpkin curry 102
    Pumpkin soup 103

quinoa
    Potato balls 73
    Swede muffins 139
—, black
    Asparagus pâté 37

red pepper
    Pom's Asian bean salad 96
    Swede ragout 140
relish
    Plum relish 121
    Rhubarb relish 28
rhubarb
    Rhubarb compote 30
    Rhubarb cordial 29
    Rhubarb relish 28
rice
    Crispbread 42
    Crustless cabbage quiche with
      spring onions 34
    Mushroom pâté 116
    —, pudding
      Rice pudding 136
rye, cracked
    Carsten's *svedjerug* bread 106

salad
    Mung bean and melon salad 69
    Pom's Asian bean salad 96
    Warm potato salad 72
sandwich spread
    Beetroot (beet) sandwich spread
      146
    Green pea sandwich spread 84
    Kale sandwich spread 151

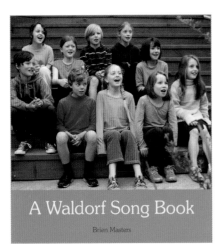

A Waldorf Song Book

Brien Masters

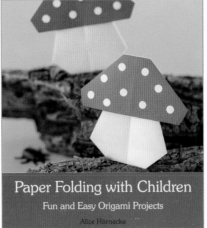

Paper Folding with Children

Fun and Easy Origami Projects

Alice Hörnecke

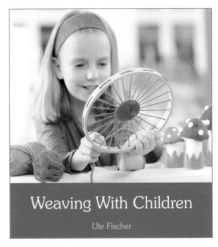

Weaving With Children

Ute Fischer

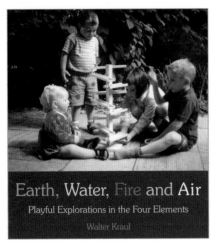

Earth, Water, Fire and Air

Playful Explorations in the Four Elements

Walter Kraul

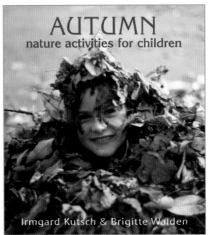

AUTUMN
nature activities for children

Irmgard Kutsch & Brigitte Walden

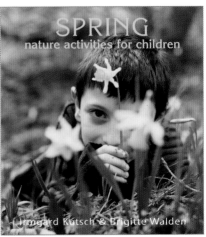

SPRING
nature activities for children

Irmgard Kutsch & Brigitte Walden

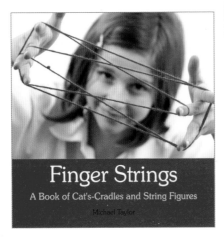

Finger Strings

A Book of Cat's-Cradles and String Figures

Michael Taylor

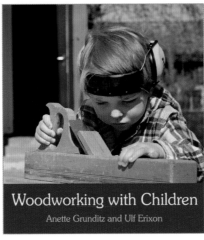

Woodworking with Children

Anette Grunditz and Ulf Erixon

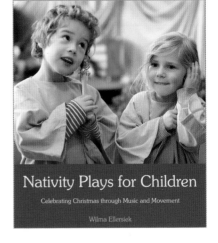

Nativity Plays for Children

Celebrating Christmas through Music and Movement

Wilma Ellersiek